CONTENTS

FOREWORD FROM CHIP
ASHLING LARKIN
PAGE 2

TAKE YOUR TIME
STORY BY NAOMI - ART BY SARA JULIA
PAGE 5

BRIGHT SMILES
STORY BY CARLY - ART BY EVE GREENWOOD
PAGE 11

REMEMBRANCE
STORY BY ANN - ART BY ELLIOT BALSON
PAGE 15

CANCER RESEARCH
STORY BY VESNA - ART BY JULES VALERA
PAGE 21

STAYING POSITIVE, KEEPING TOGETHER
STORY BY RAJ - ART BY CATRIONA LAIRD
PAGE 26

GREY MATTERS
STORY BY WALKIRIA LARKIN - ART BY ASHLING LARKIN
PAGE 32

THE STORY OF CHIP
CATRIONA LAIRD
PAGE 36

CONTRIBUTOR LIST
PAGE 38

THE MAKING OF THE COMICS
PAGE 40

KICKSTARTER BACKERS
PAGE 42

FOREWORD FROM CHIP

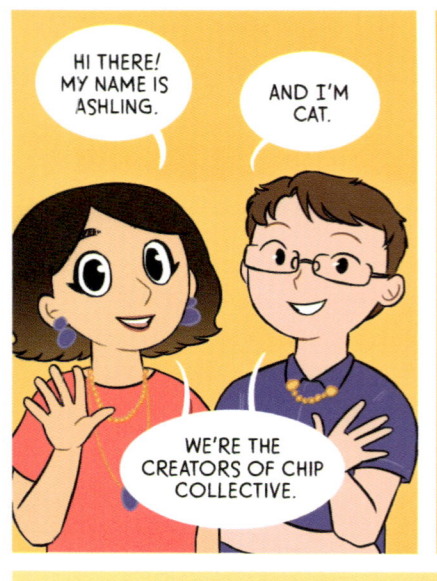
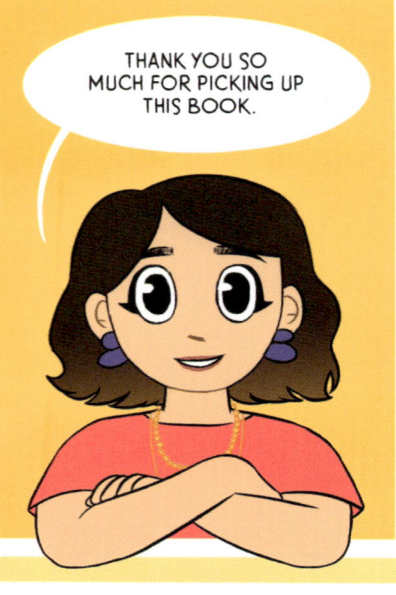
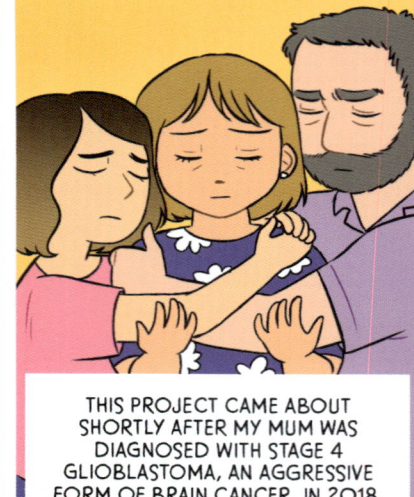

Living with Cancer
OUR STORIES

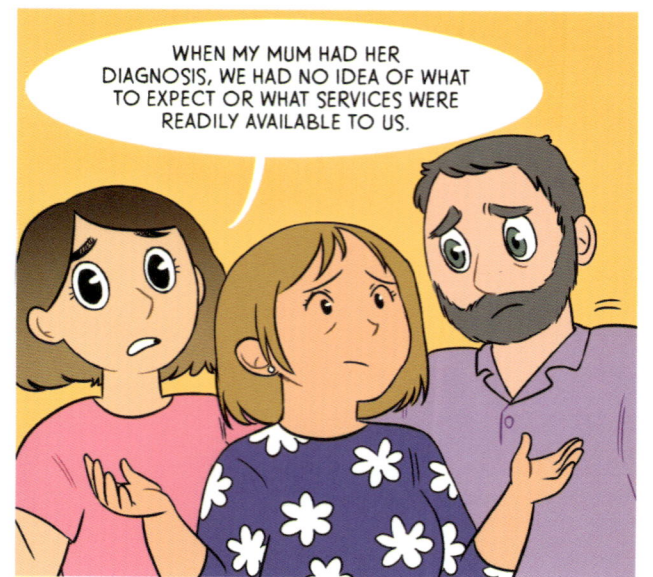
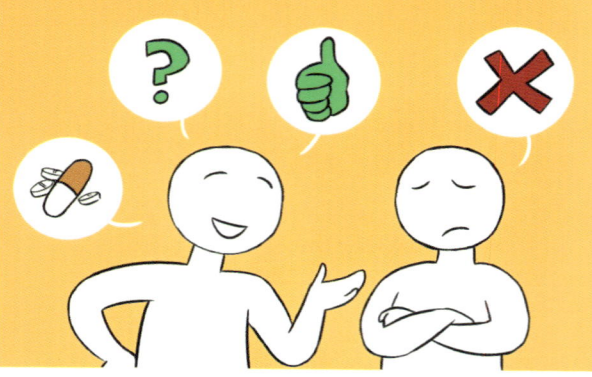

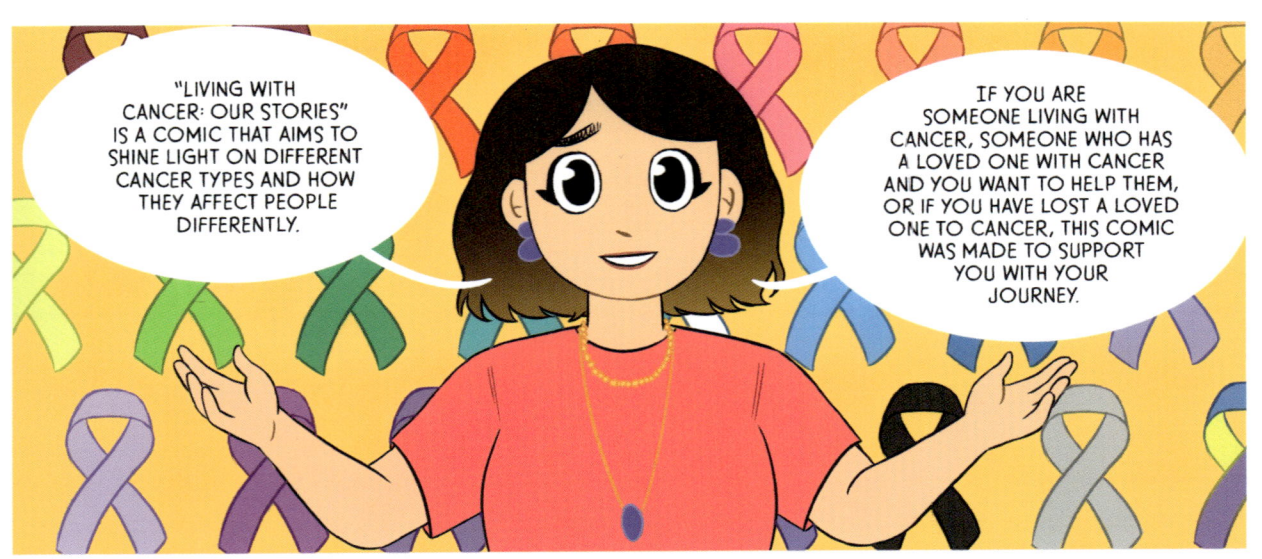

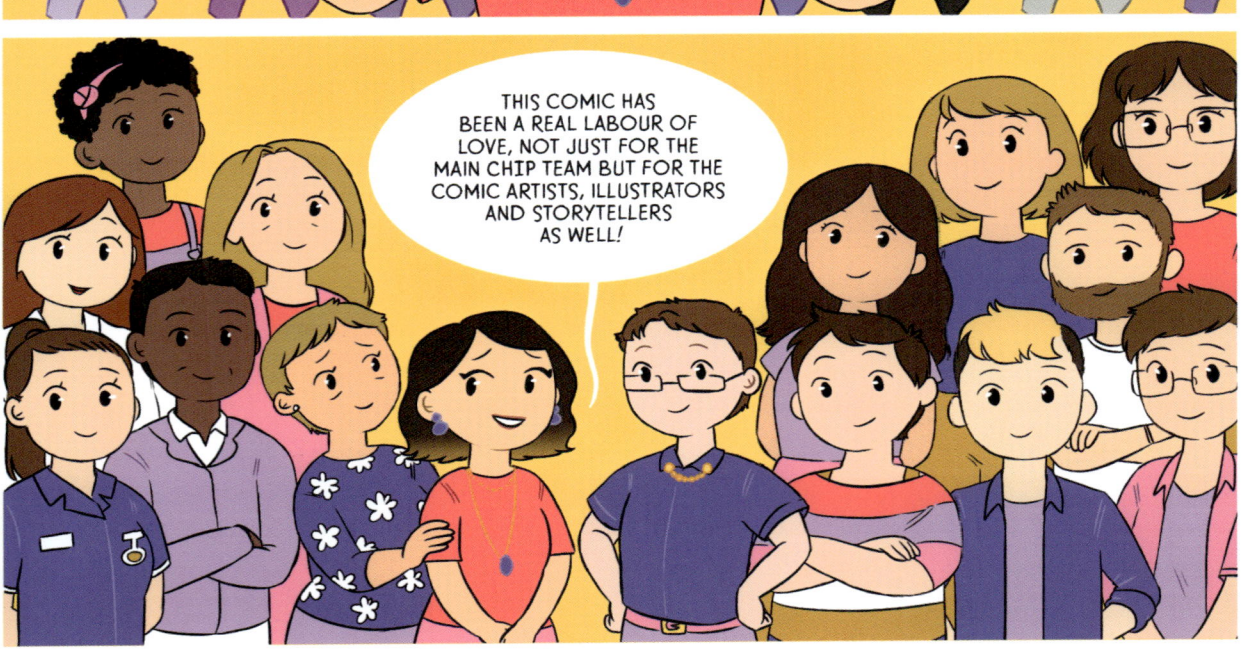

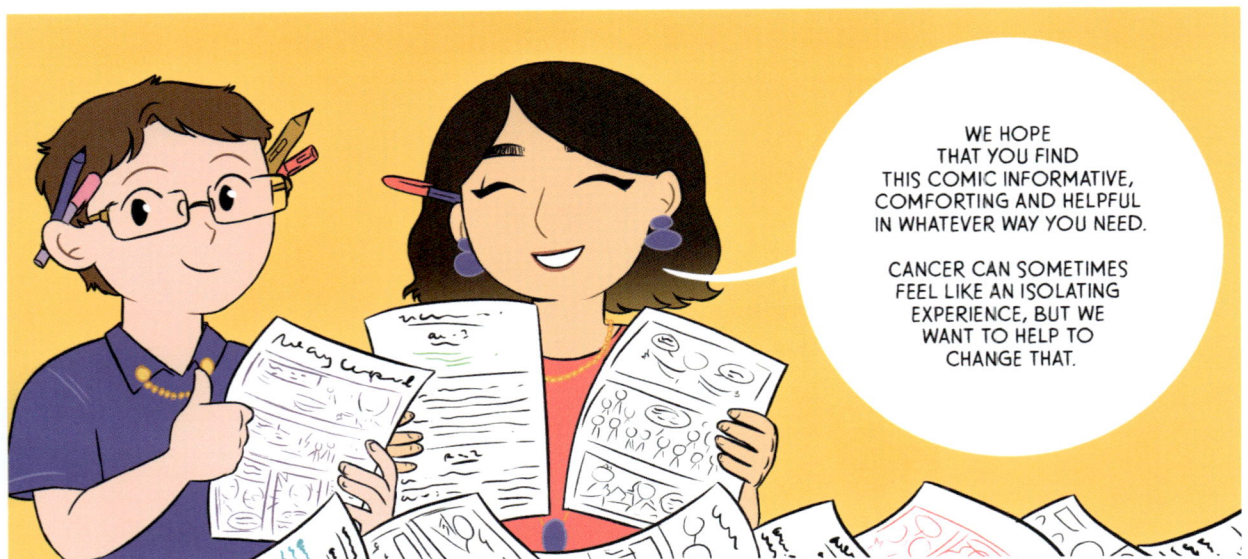

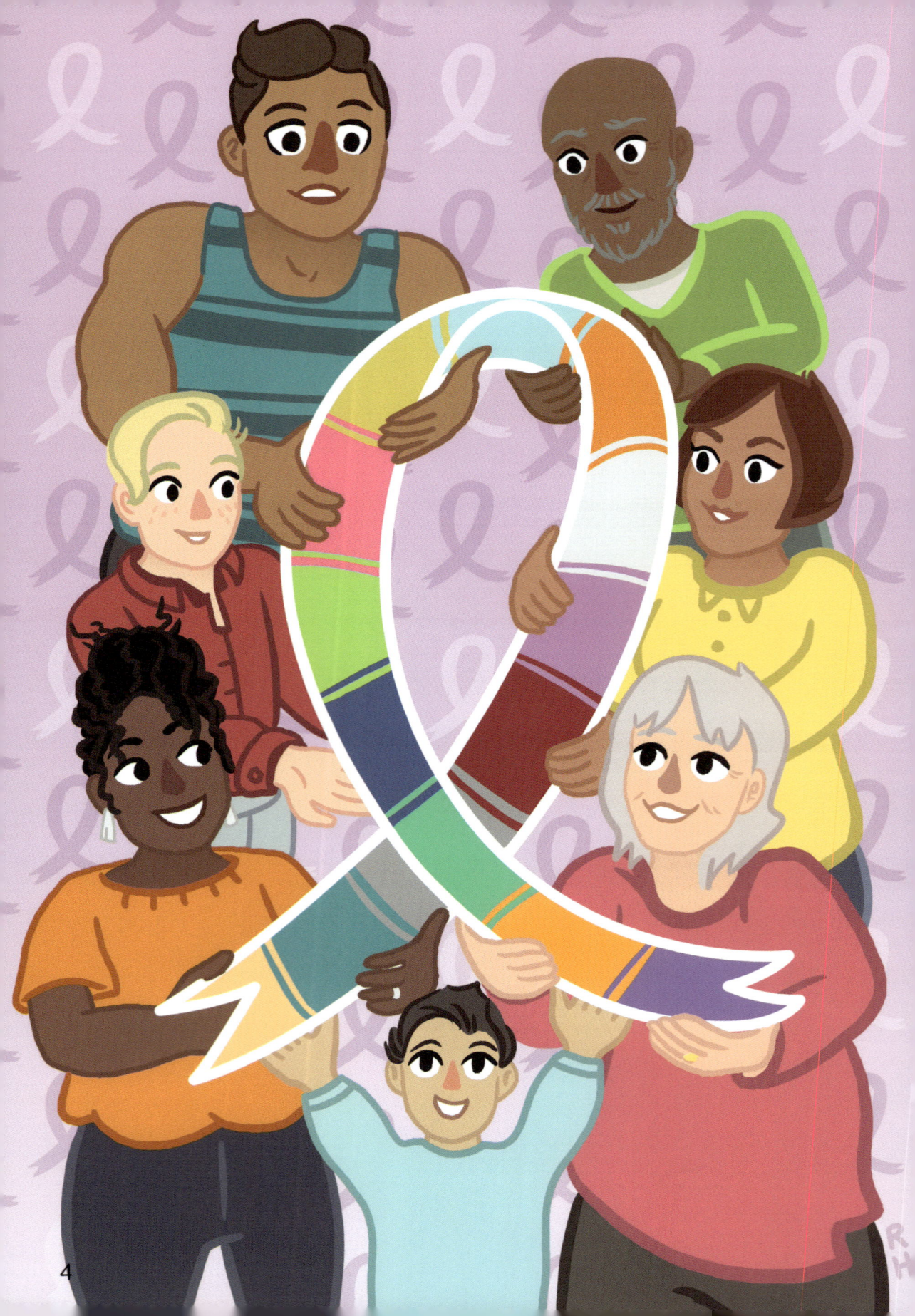

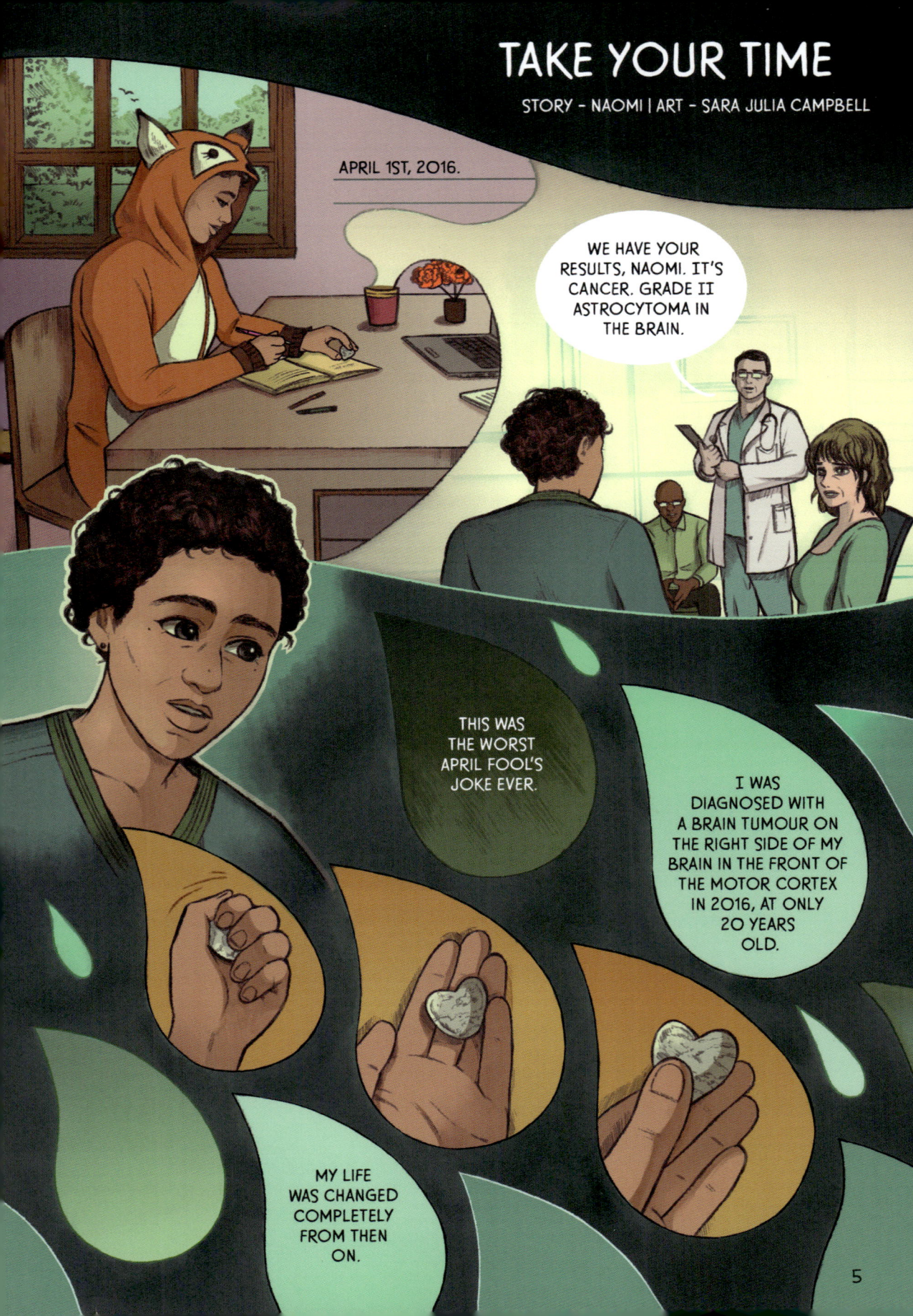

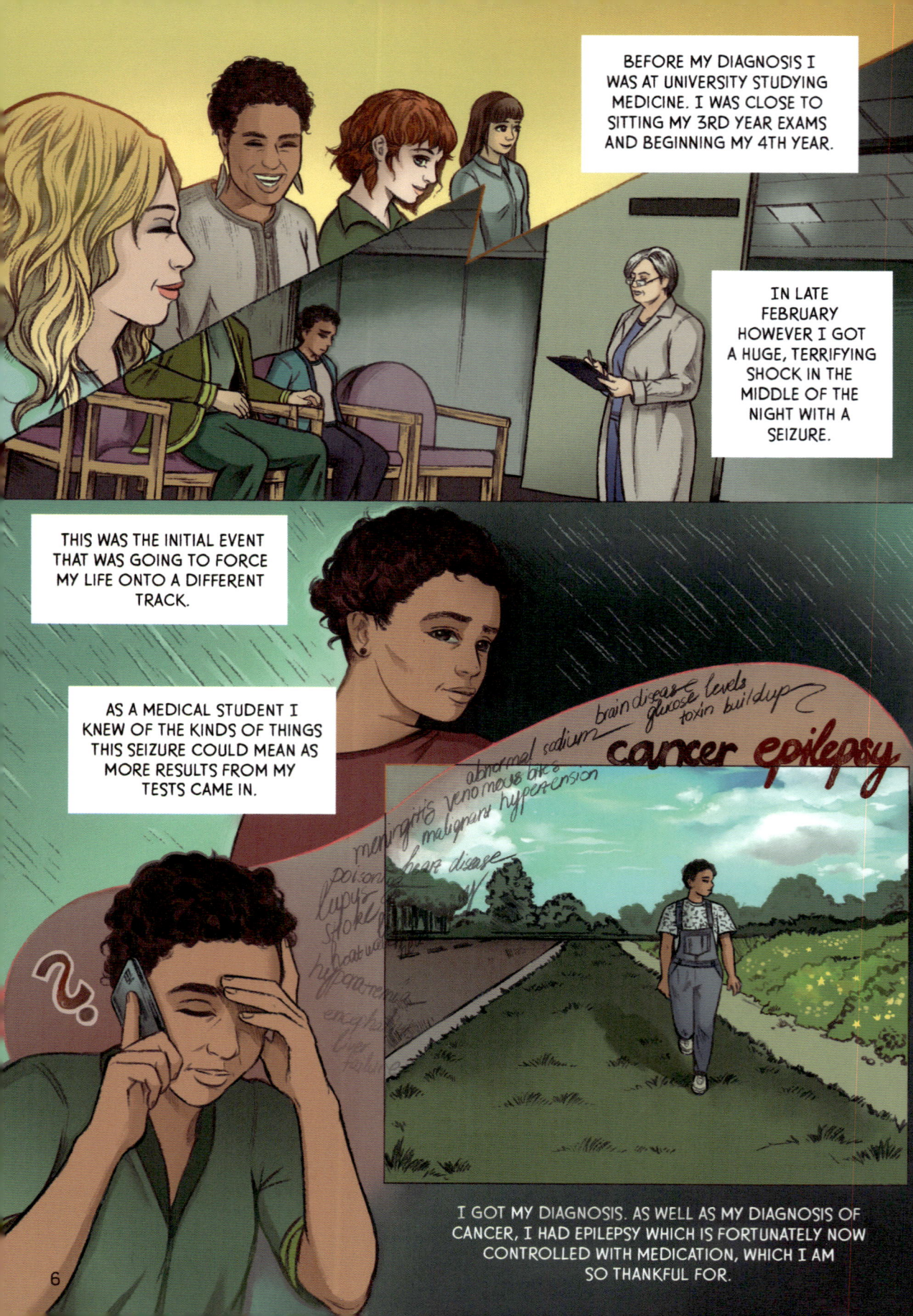

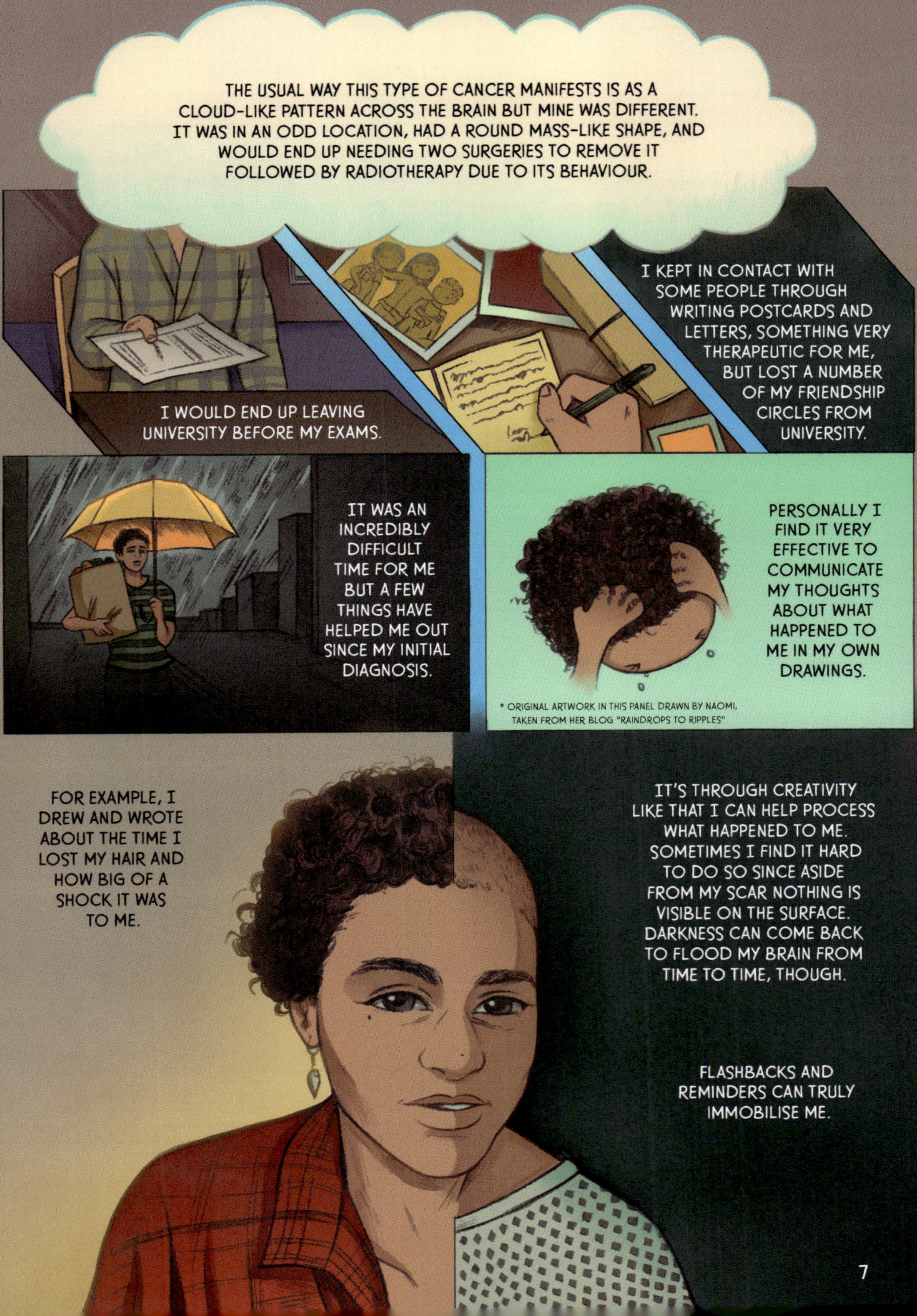

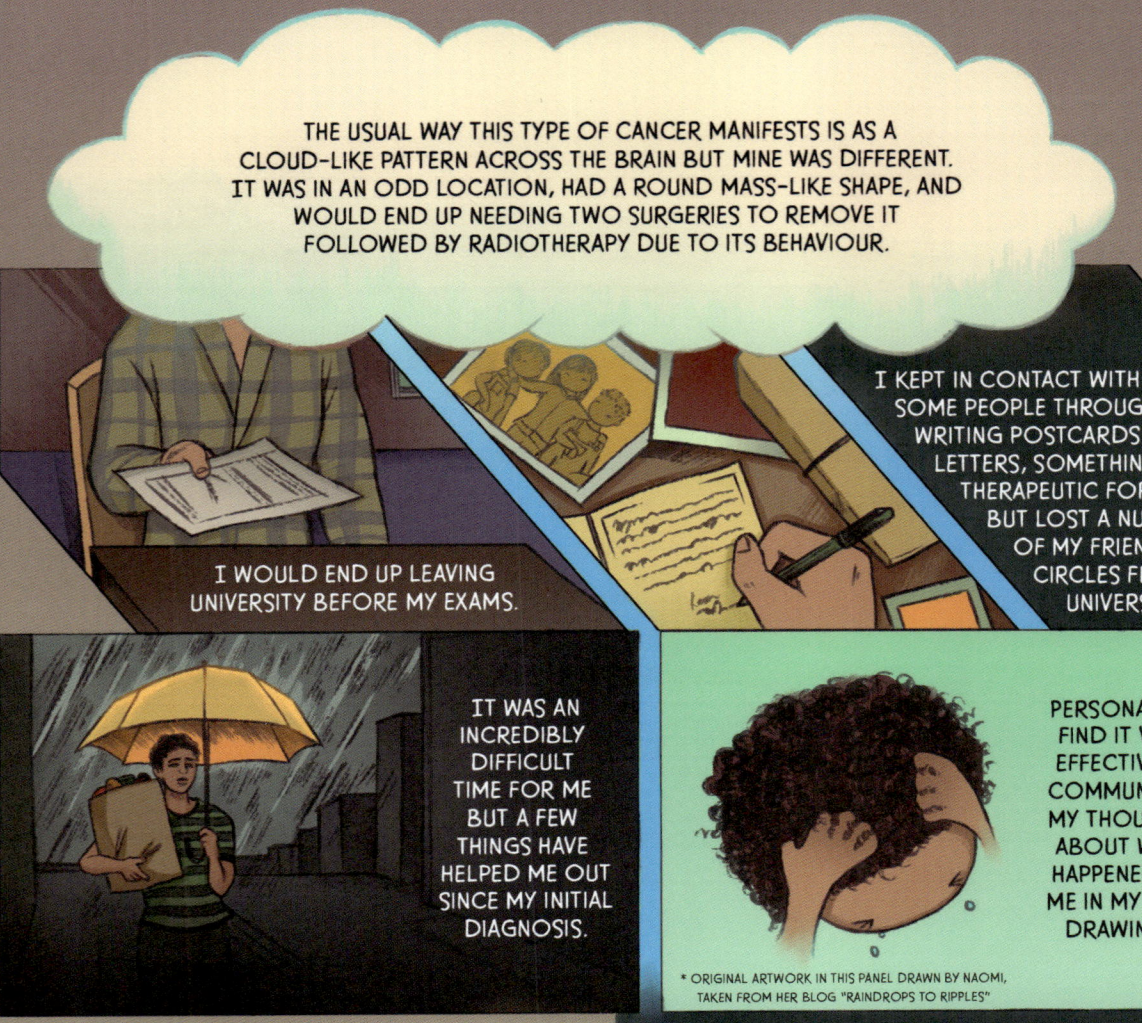

I'VE BEEN HELPED BY SO MANY DIFFERENT PEOPLE AND ORGANISATIONS IN DIFFERENT WAYS. THEY ARE ALL WONDERFULLY COMPASSIONATE AND HAVE NOT ONLY LISTENED TO ME BUT *HEARD* ME.

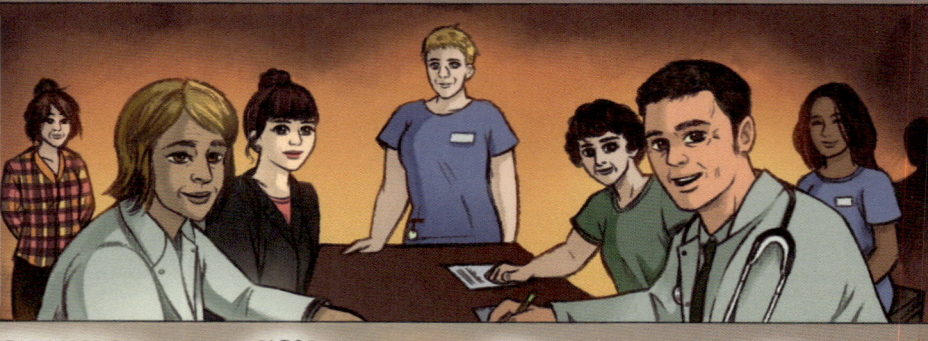

THE WILLOW FOUNDATION CHARITY.

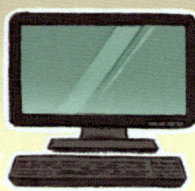

HI NAOMI, HOW DOES CIRCE DU SOLEIL SOUND? I THINK THAT WOULD BE A GREAT TRIP TO KEEP YOU GOING! BEST WISHES,

ART THERAPY SESSIONS WITH DONNA WHILE MY RADIOTHERAPY WAS ONGOING.

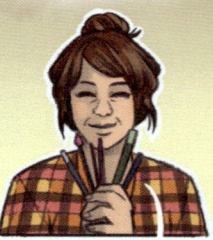

YOUR ARTWORK IS COMING ALONG GREAT, KEEP IT UP!

CLICC SARGENT.

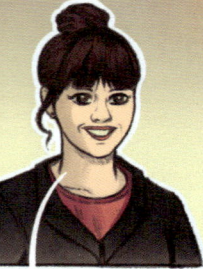

WE'VE GOT A GRANT OR SOCIAL CARE SUPPORT ORGANISED FOR YOU IF YOU DECIDE YOU NEED IT.

TEENAGE CANCER TRUST NURSES (TCT).

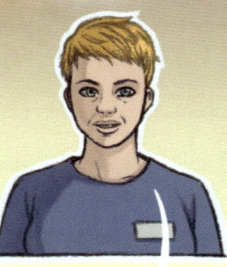

HOW DO YOU FEEL TODAY? CAN I HELP?

AND MY FRIEND ABI.

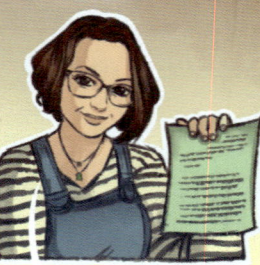

HEY, NAOMI, CHECK OUT THIS ARTICLE I FOUND, I THOUGHT YOU MIGHT ENJOY IT!

AT FIRST I ACTIVELY CHOSE NOT TO ASSOCIATE WITH CANCER PATIENTS OR SURVIVORS AFTER MY DIAGNOSIS. IT WAS ONLY IN 2018 I DECIDED TO REALLY GET INVOLVED WITH TCT EVENTS AND NOW I HAVE ABI TO TALK TO.

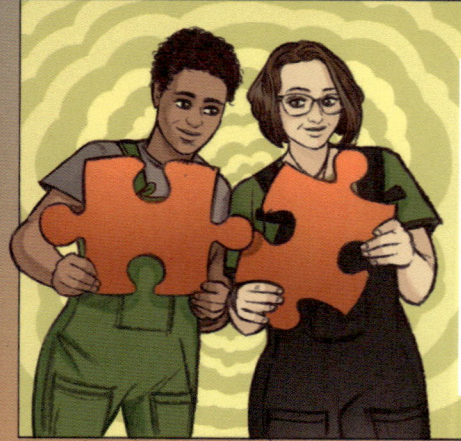

WE DON'T NEED TO TALK ABOUT CANCER TOGETHER, IT'S THE COMFORT IN KNOWING WHAT WE'VE BOTH BEEN THROUGH AND KNOWING WE CAN TALK IN A DIFFERENT WAY WITH EACH OTHER THAN WE CAN WITH OTHER PEOPLE THAT TRULY MAKES OUR FRIENDSHIP SPECIAL.

WITH PEOPLE IN GENERAL THERE ARE PEOPLE YOU CLICK WITH AND PEOPLE YOU DON'T. SOMETIMES IN TCT EVENTS I FEEL IT'S AN ASSUMED GIVEN THAT YOU WILL SHARE YOUR STORY AND BE FRIENDS WITH EVERYONE BUT THAT'S NOT THE CASE. ABI AND I JUST CLICK.

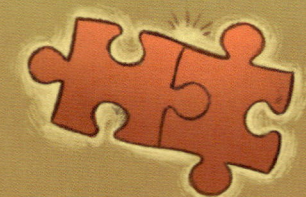

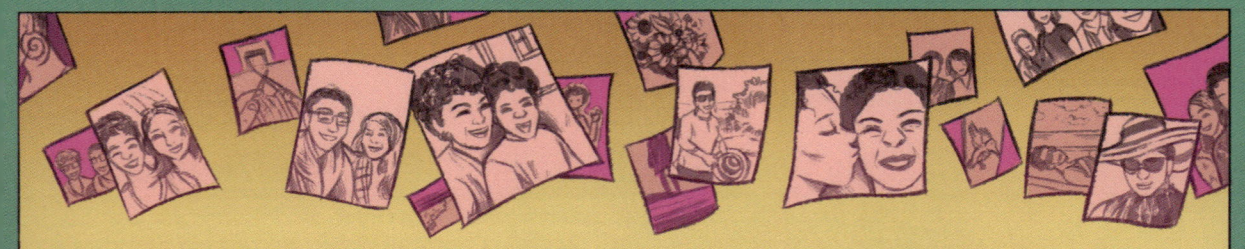

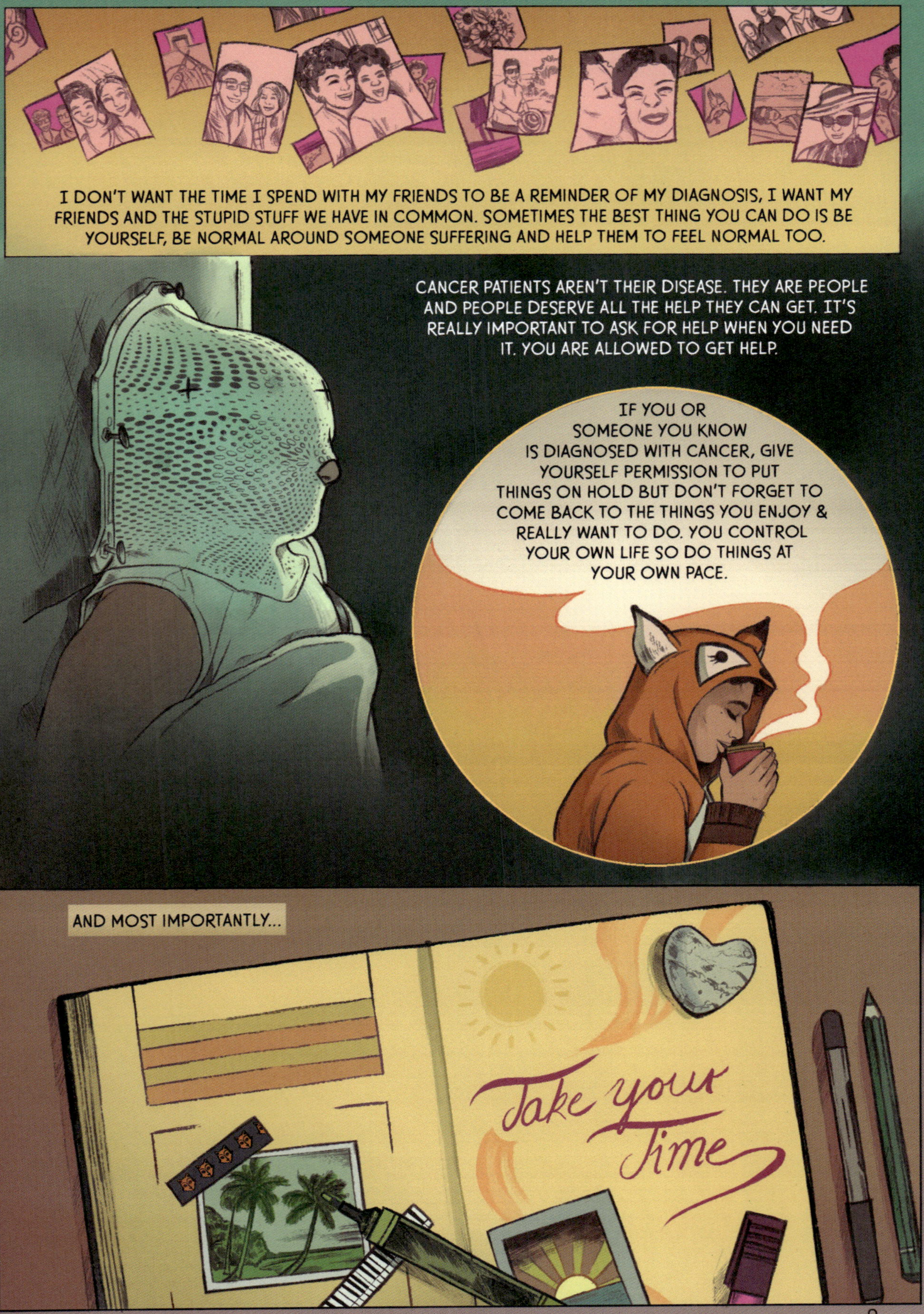

I DON'T WANT THE TIME I SPEND WITH MY FRIENDS TO BE A REMINDER OF MY DIAGNOSIS, I WANT MY FRIENDS AND THE STUPID STUFF WE HAVE IN COMMON. SOMETIMES THE BEST THING YOU CAN DO IS BE YOURSELF, BE NORMAL AROUND SOMEONE SUFFERING AND HELP THEM TO FEEL NORMAL TOO.

CANCER PATIENTS AREN'T THEIR DISEASE. THEY ARE PEOPLE AND PEOPLE DESERVE ALL THE HELP THEY CAN GET. IT'S REALLY IMPORTANT TO ASK FOR HELP WHEN YOU NEED IT. YOU ARE ALLOWED TO GET HELP.

IF YOU OR SOMEONE YOU KNOW IS DIAGNOSED WITH CANCER, GIVE YOURSELF PERMISSION TO PUT THINGS ON HOLD BUT DON'T FORGET TO COME BACK TO THE THINGS YOU ENJOY & REALLY WANT TO DO. YOU CONTROL YOUR OWN LIFE SO DO THINGS AT YOUR OWN PACE.

AND MOST IMPORTANTLY...

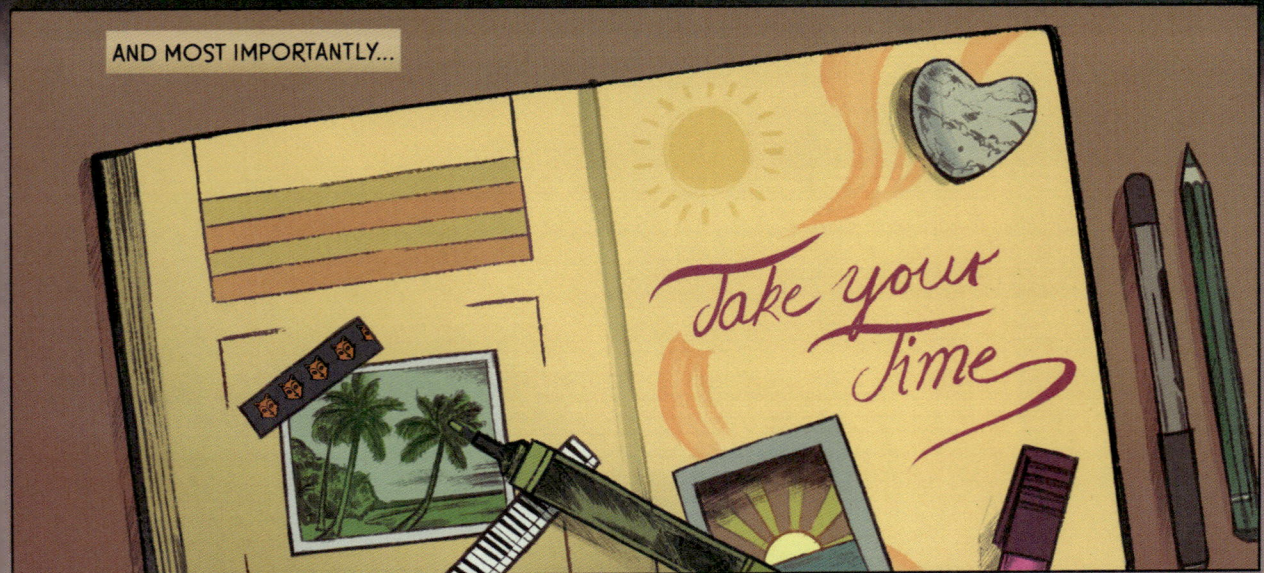

Take your Time

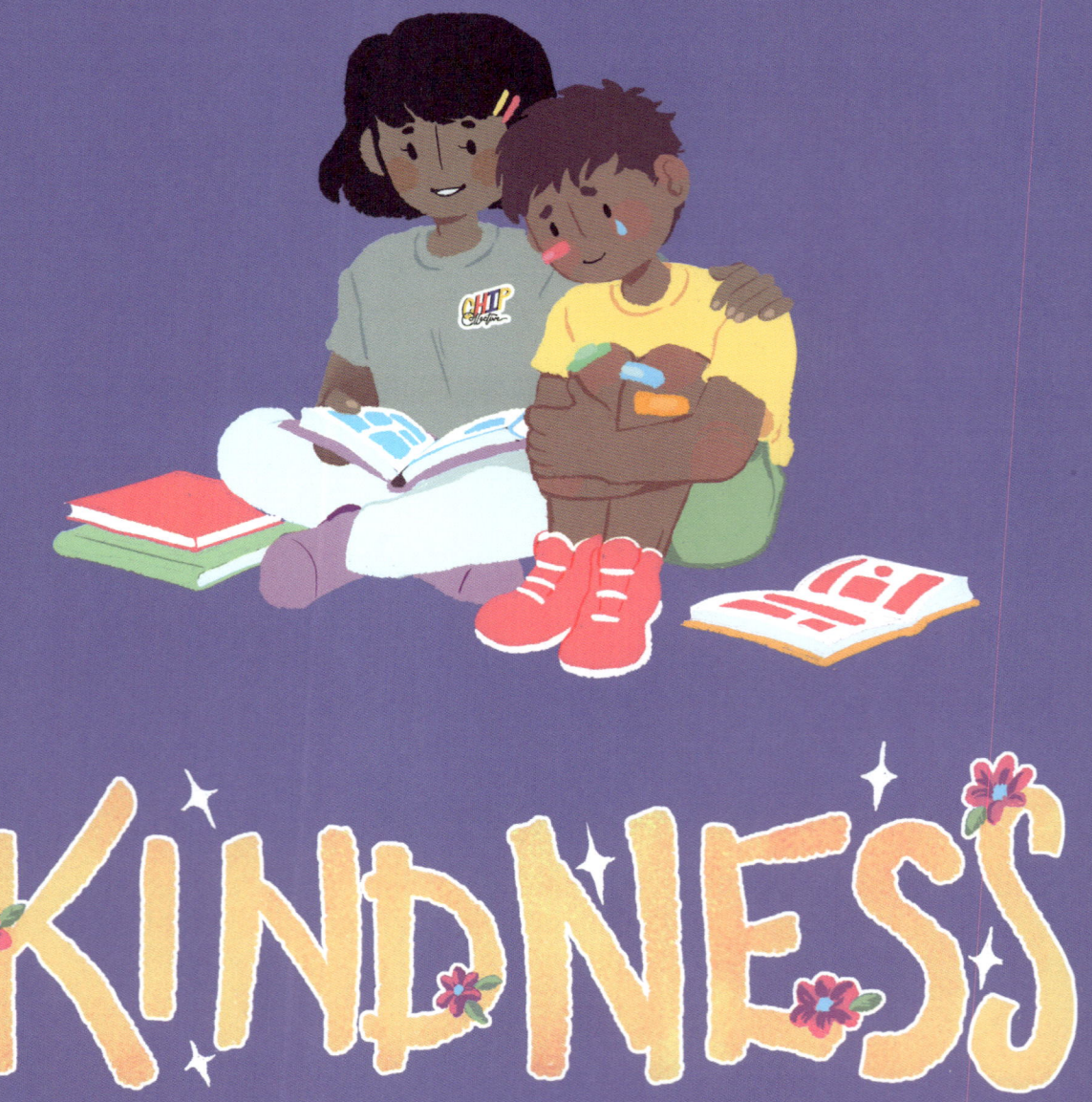

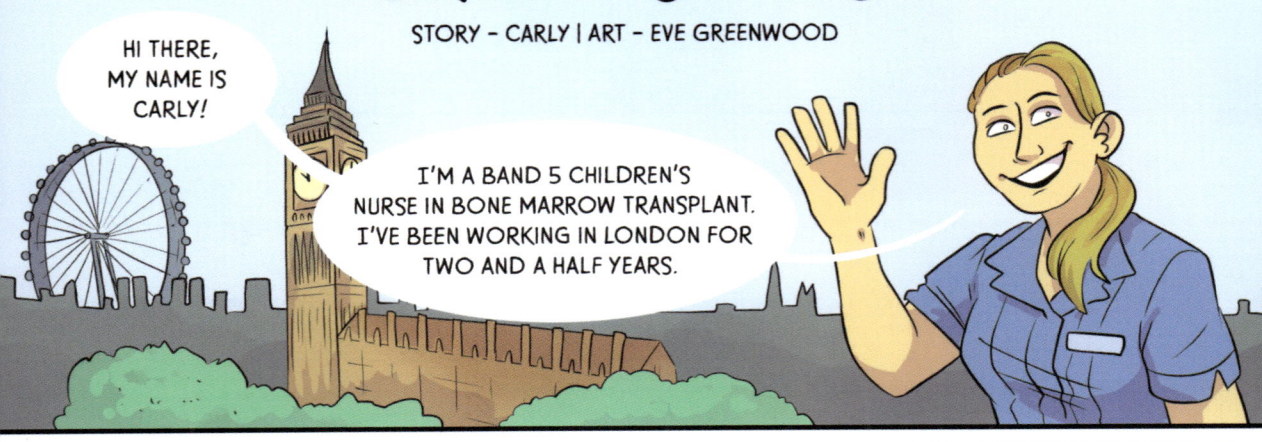

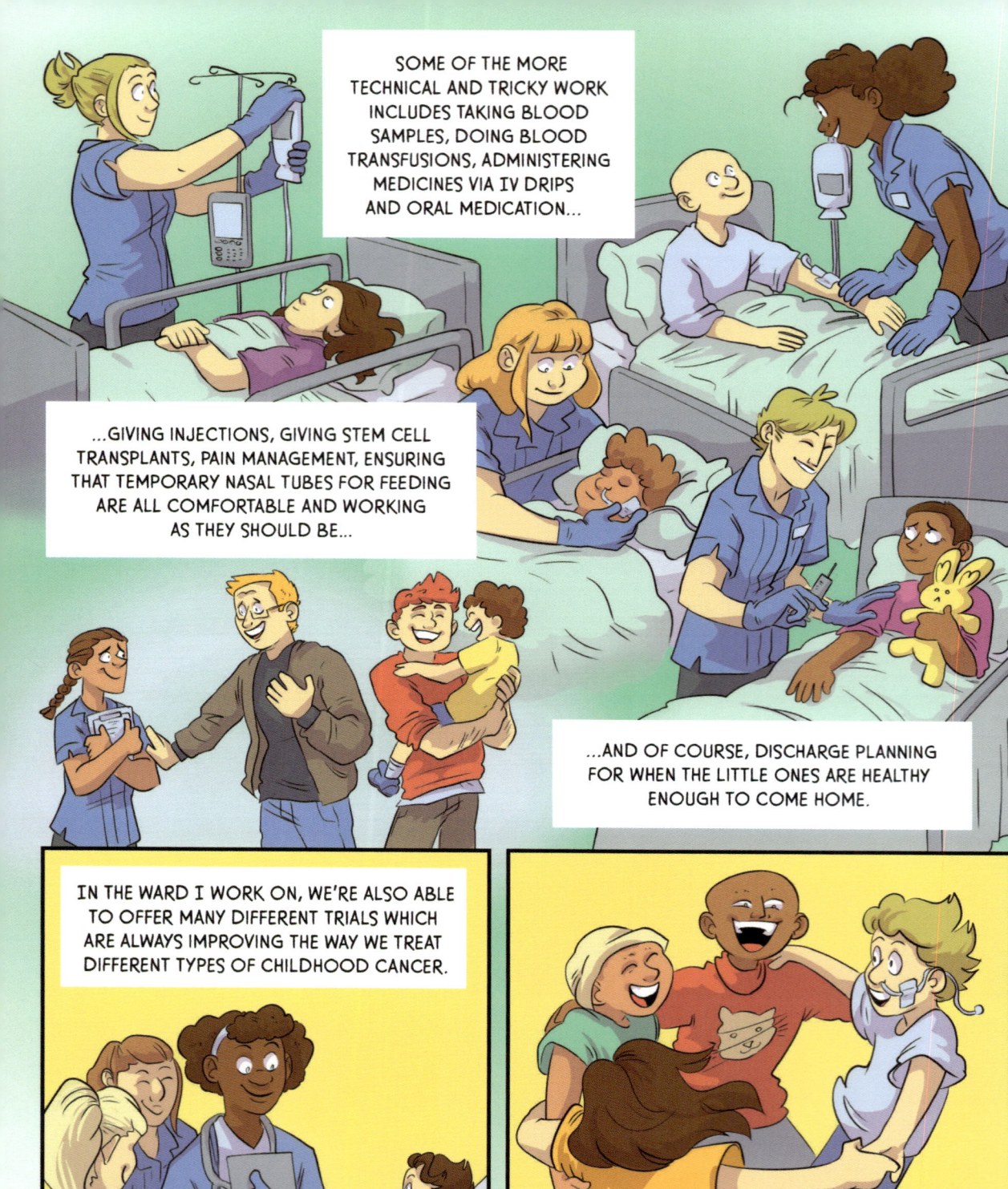

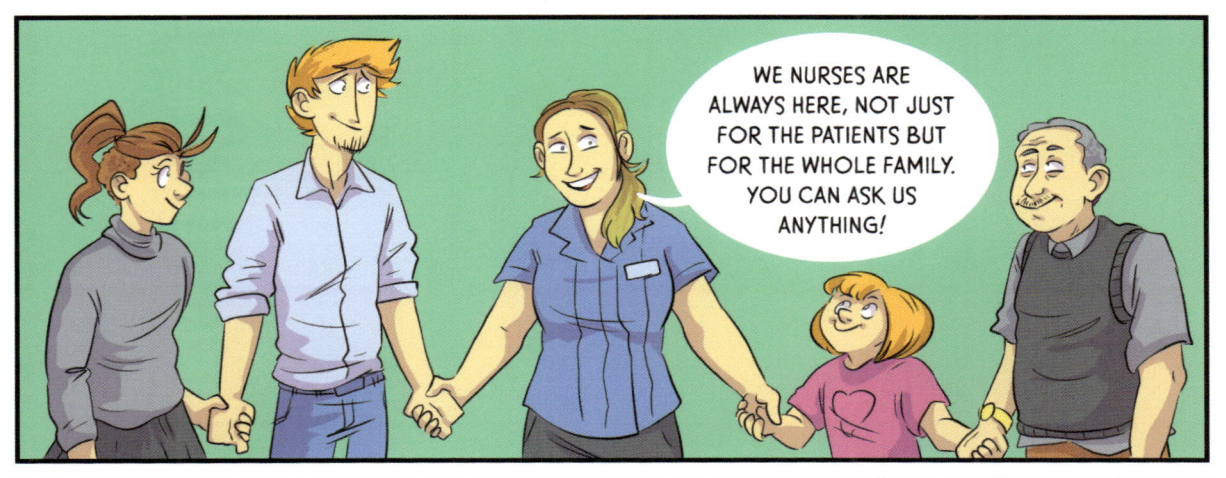
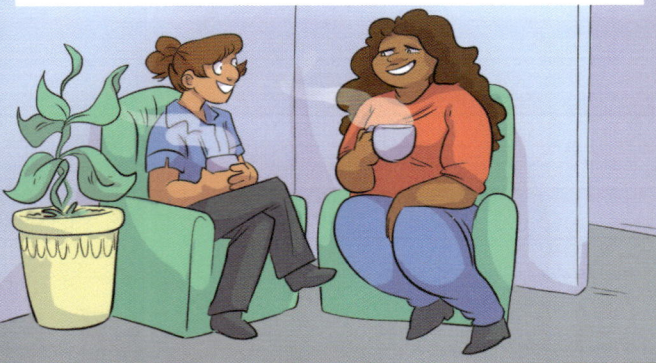
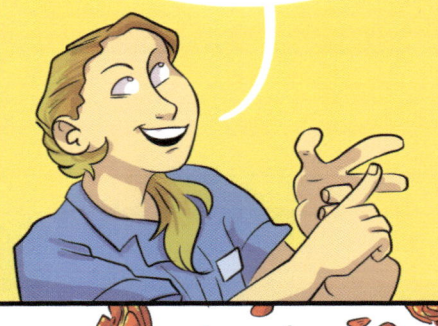
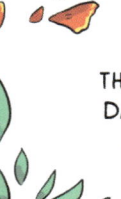
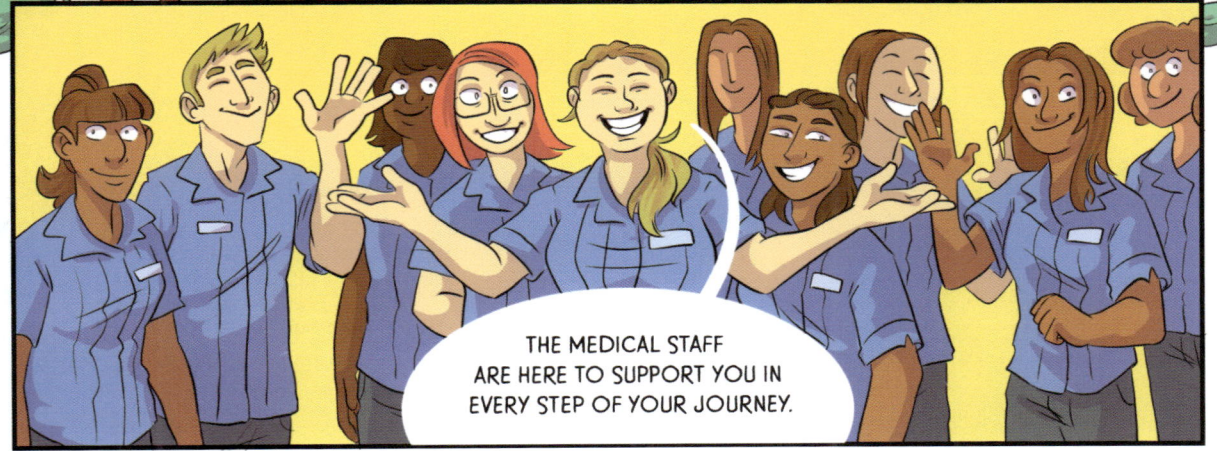

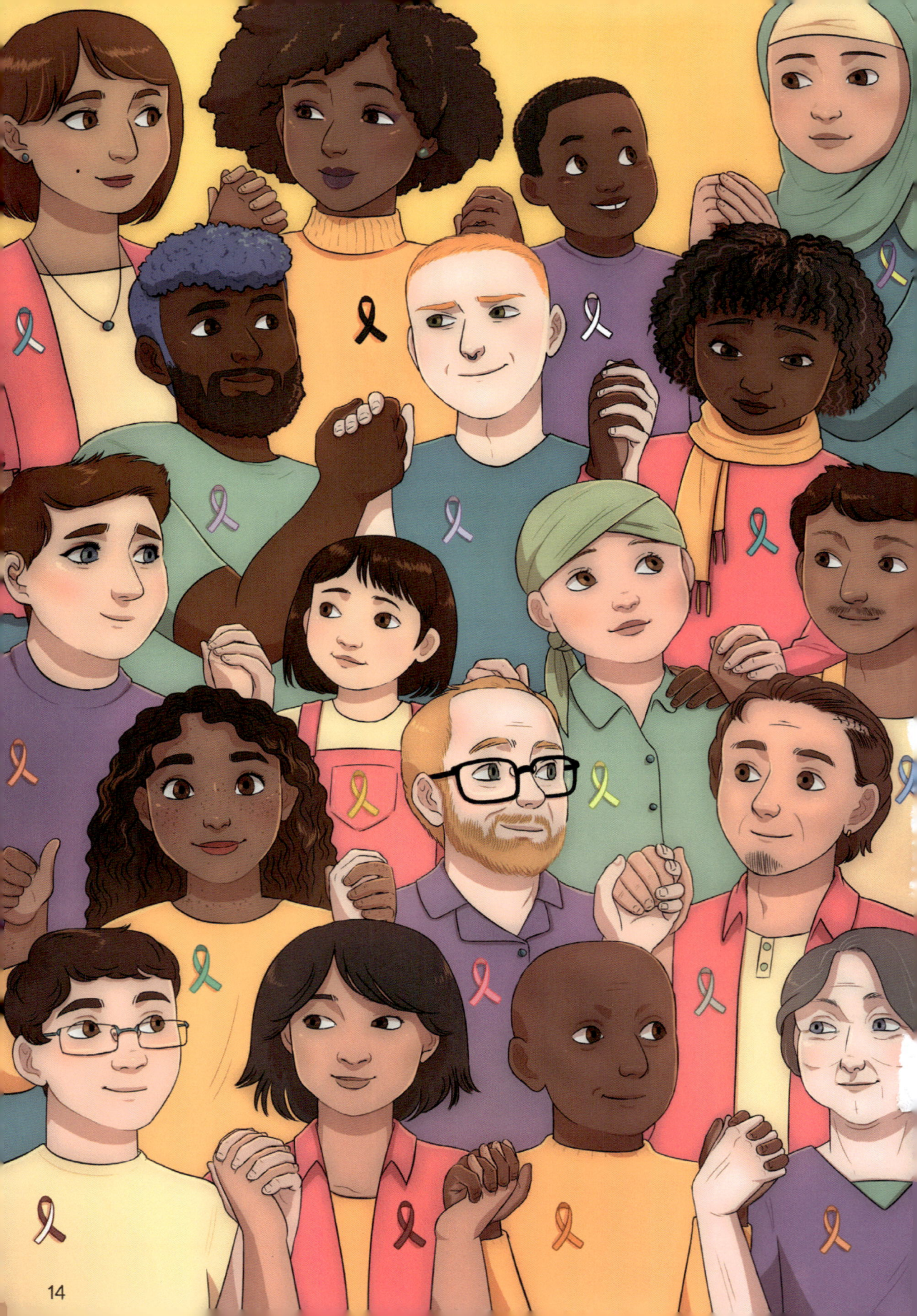

REMEMBRANCE

STORY - ANN | ART - ELLIOT BALSON

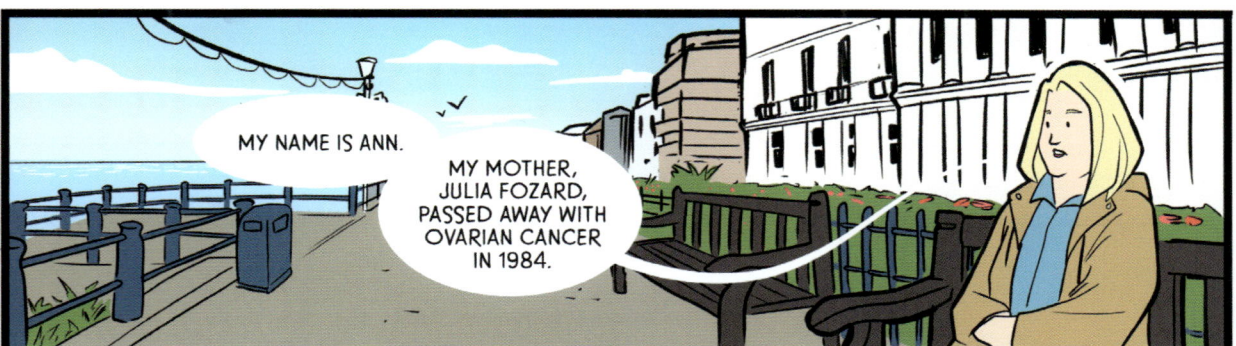

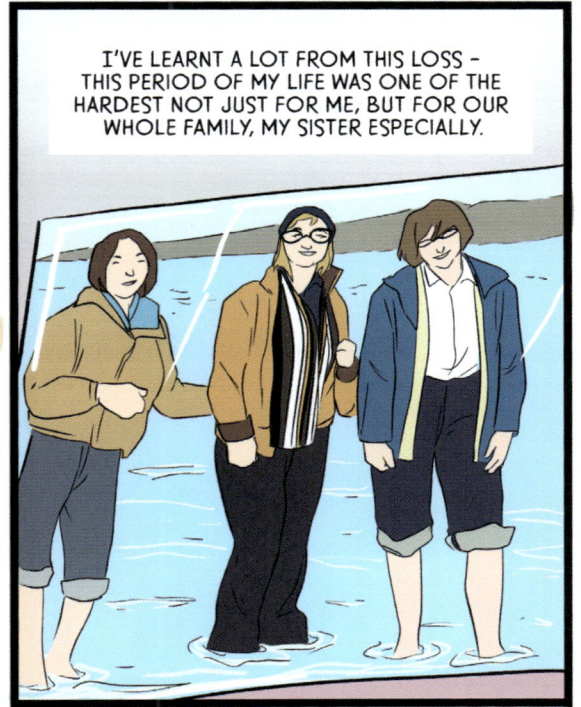

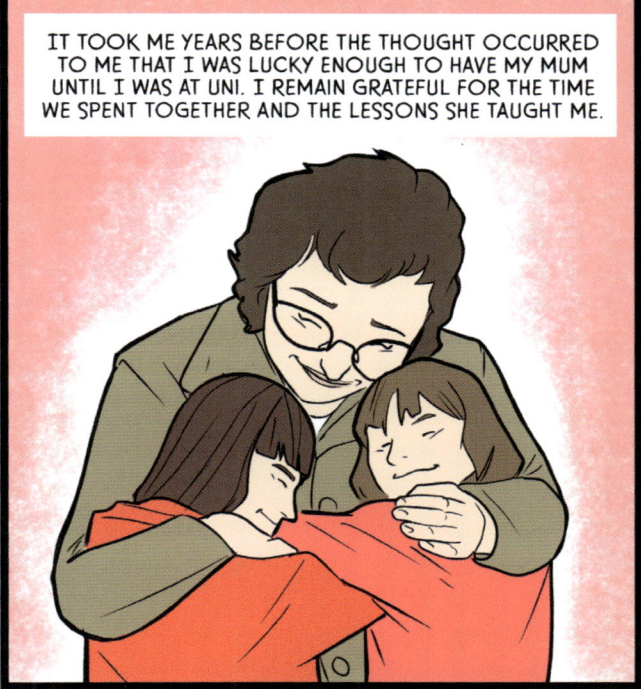

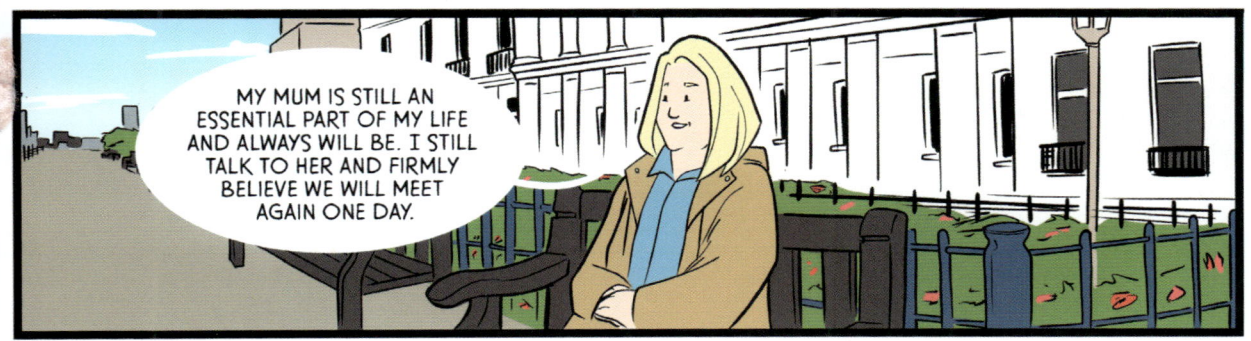

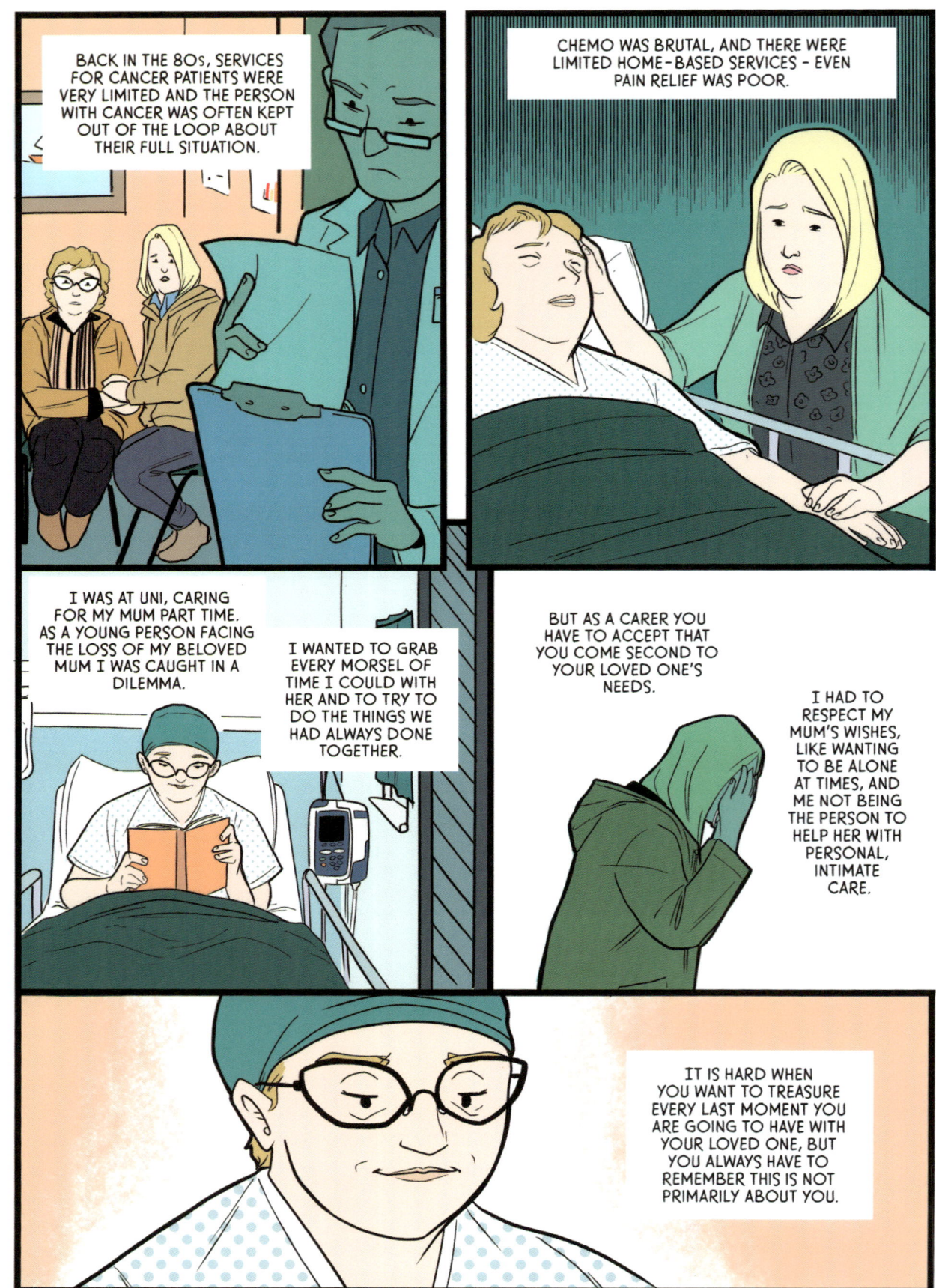

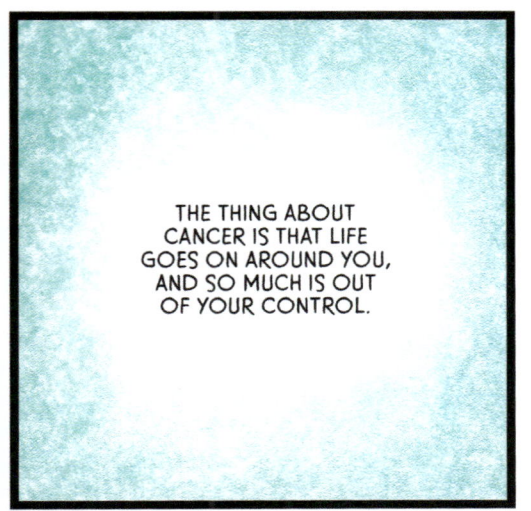
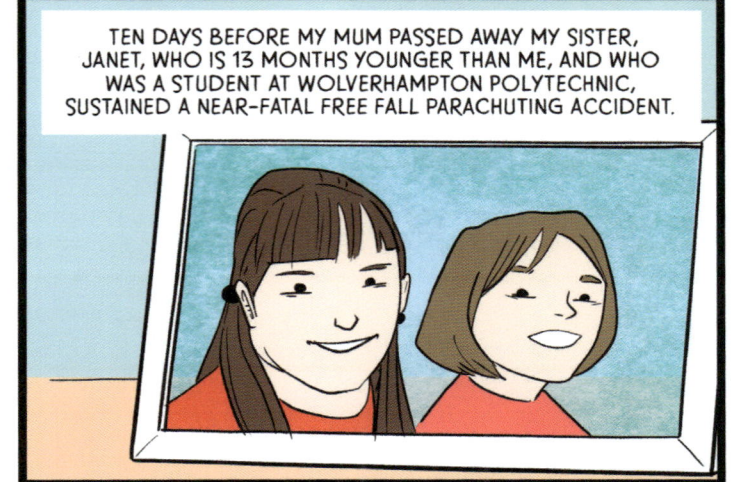
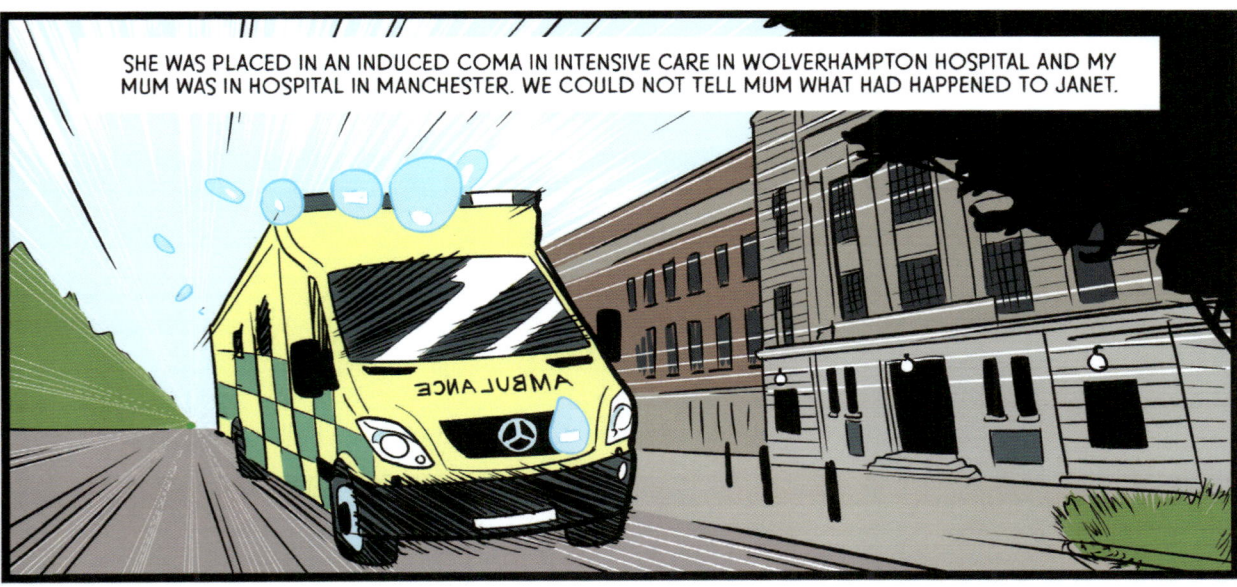
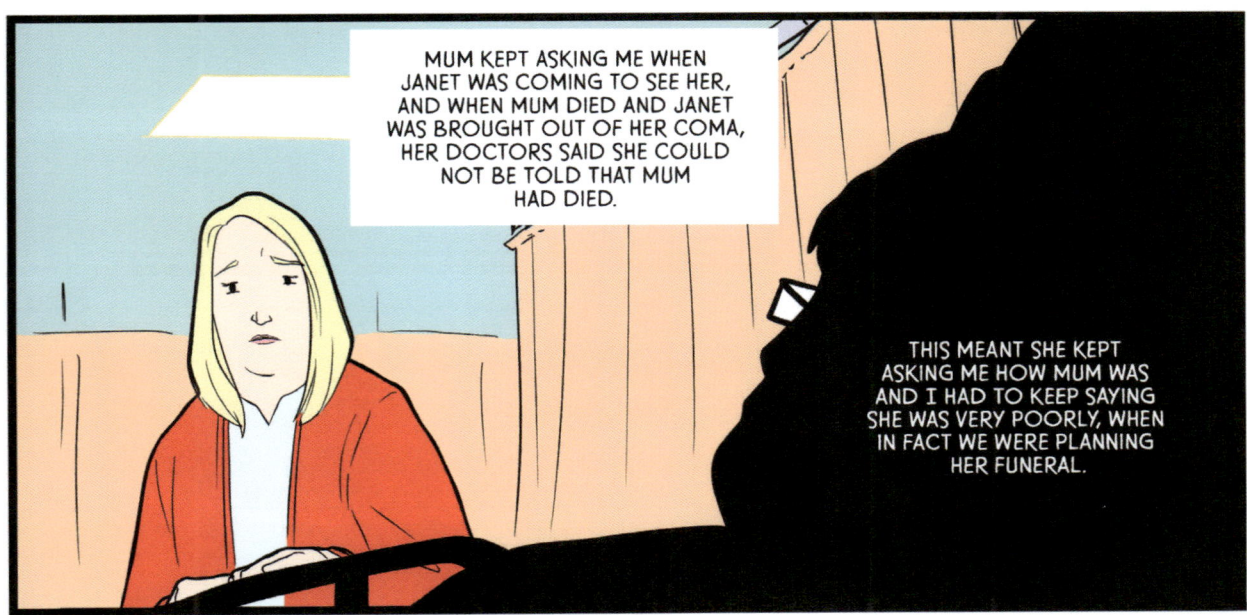

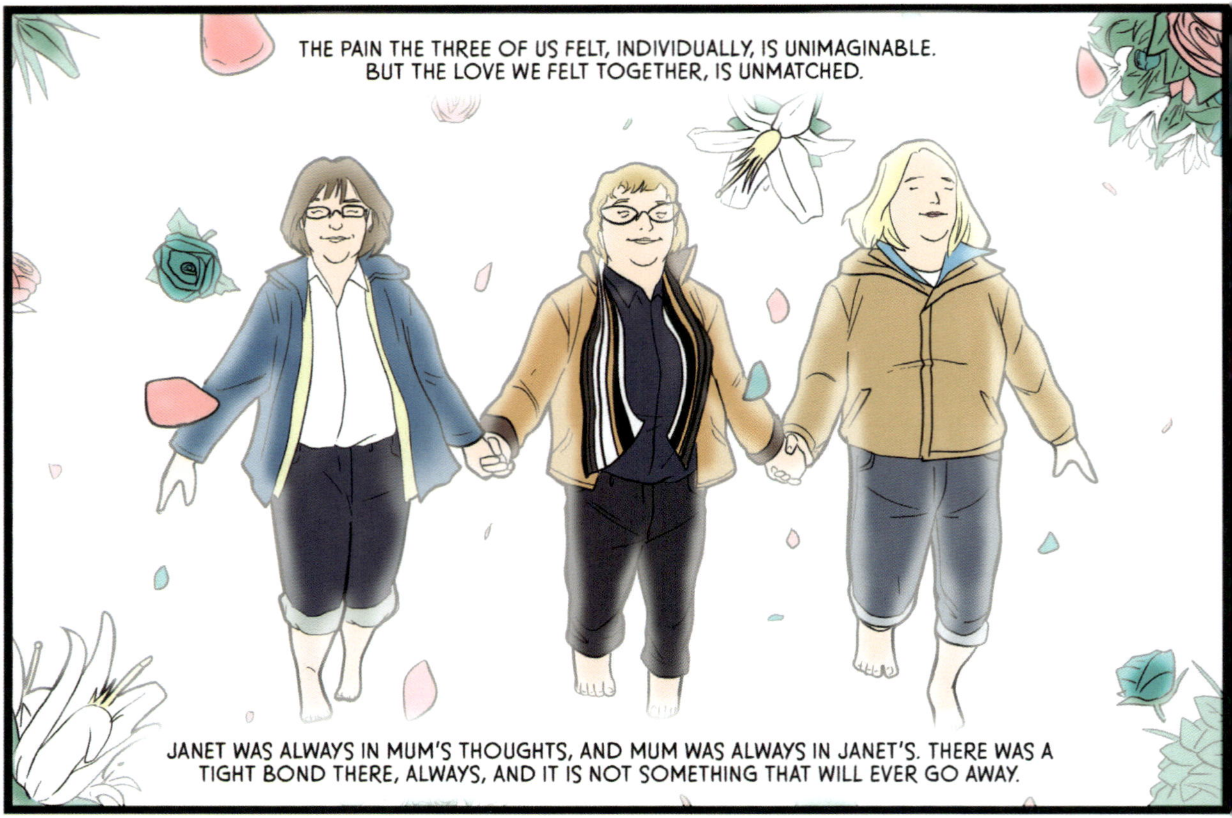

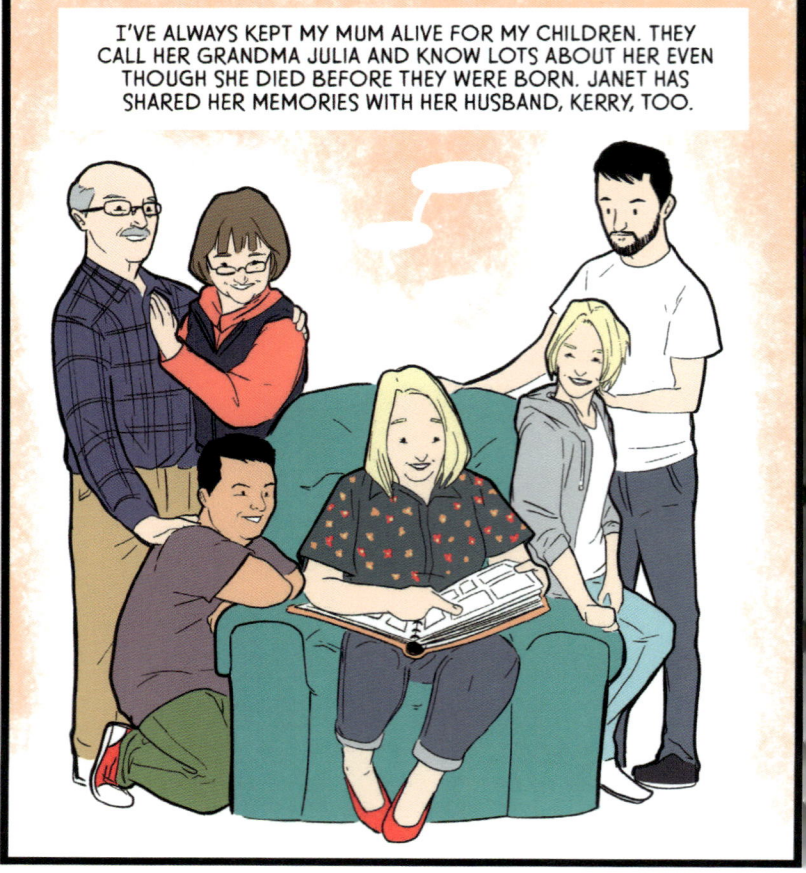

THE PAIN THE THREE OF US FELT, INDIVIDUALLY, IS UNIMAGINABLE. BUT THE LOVE WE FELT TOGETHER, IS UNMATCHED.

JANET WAS ALWAYS IN MUM'S THOUGHTS, AND MUM WAS ALWAYS IN JANET'S. THERE WAS A TIGHT BOND THERE, ALWAYS, AND IT IS NOT SOMETHING THAT WILL EVER GO AWAY.

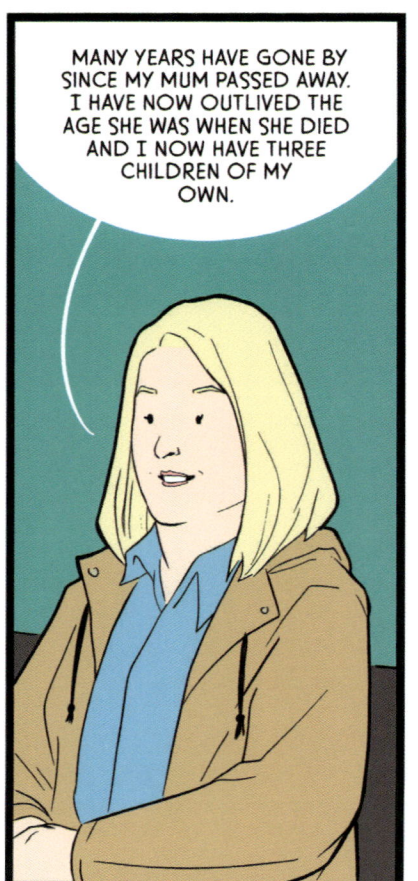

MANY YEARS HAVE GONE BY SINCE MY MUM PASSED AWAY. I HAVE NOW OUTLIVED THE AGE SHE WAS WHEN SHE DIED AND I NOW HAVE THREE CHILDREN OF MY OWN.

I'VE ALWAYS KEPT MY MUM ALIVE FOR MY CHILDREN. THEY CALL HER GRANDMA JULIA AND KNOW LOTS ABOUT HER EVEN THOUGH SHE DIED BEFORE THEY WERE BORN. JANET HAS SHARED HER MEMORIES WITH HER HUSBAND, KERRY, TOO.

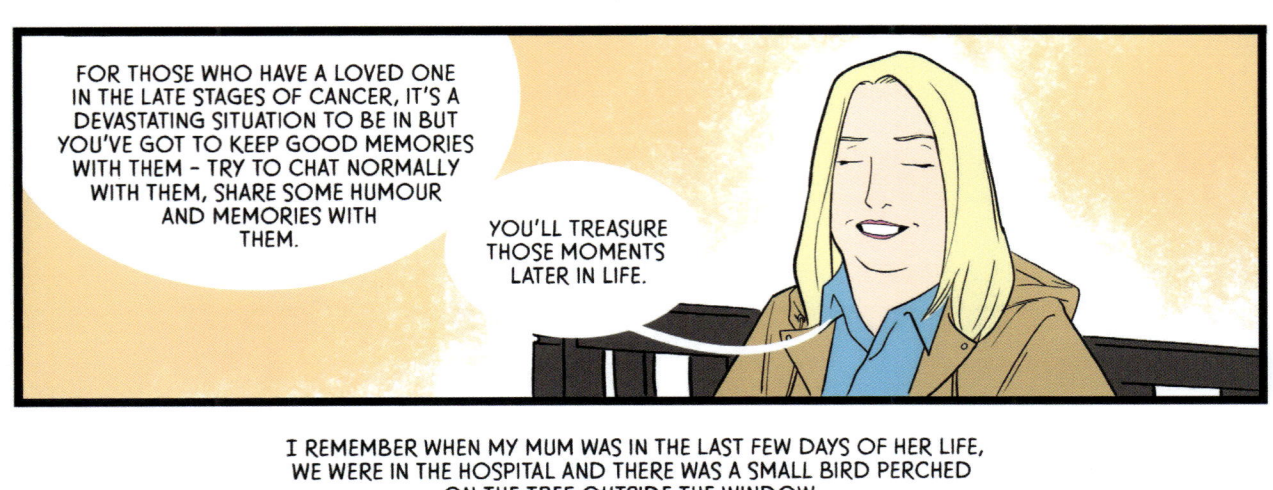

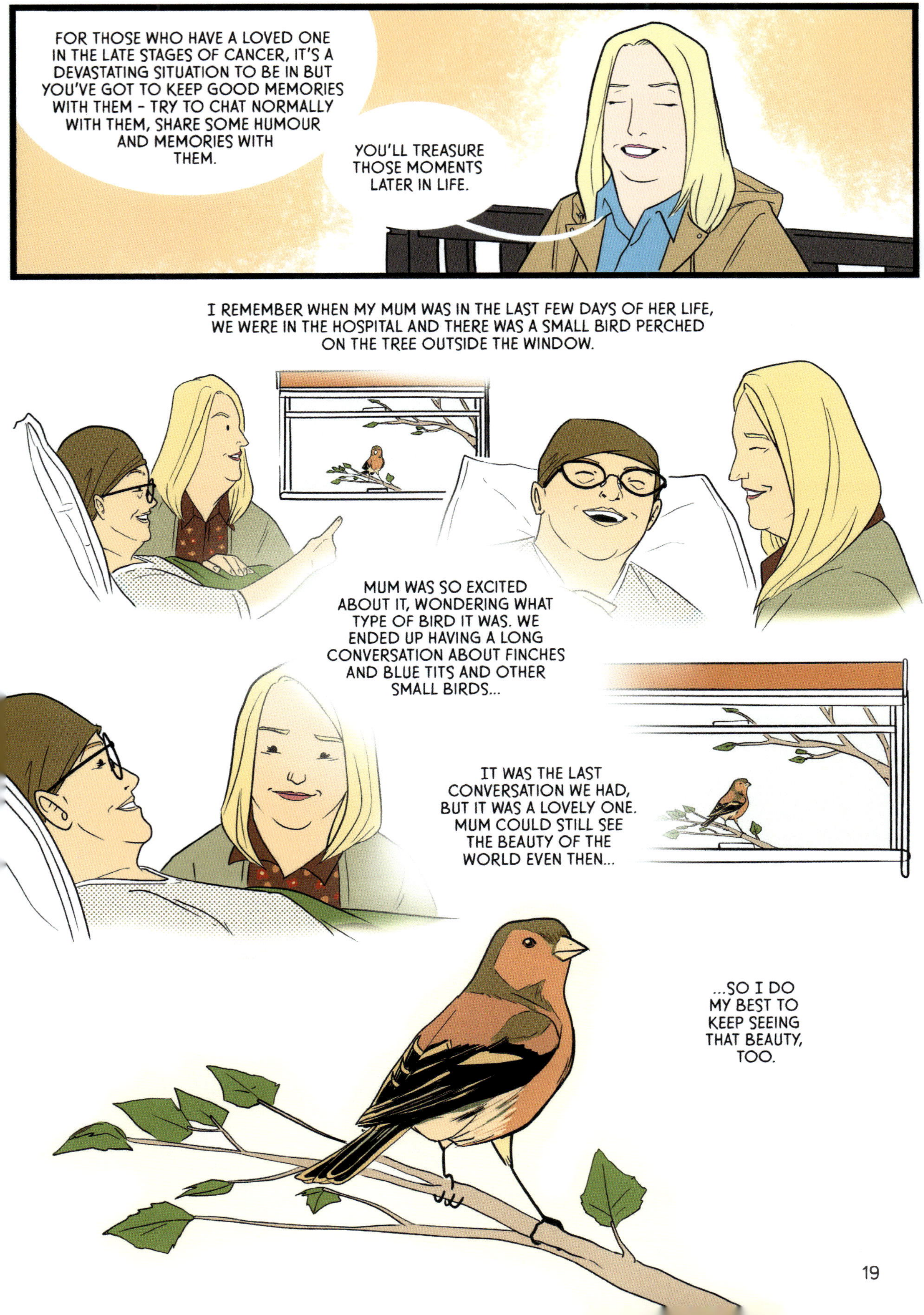

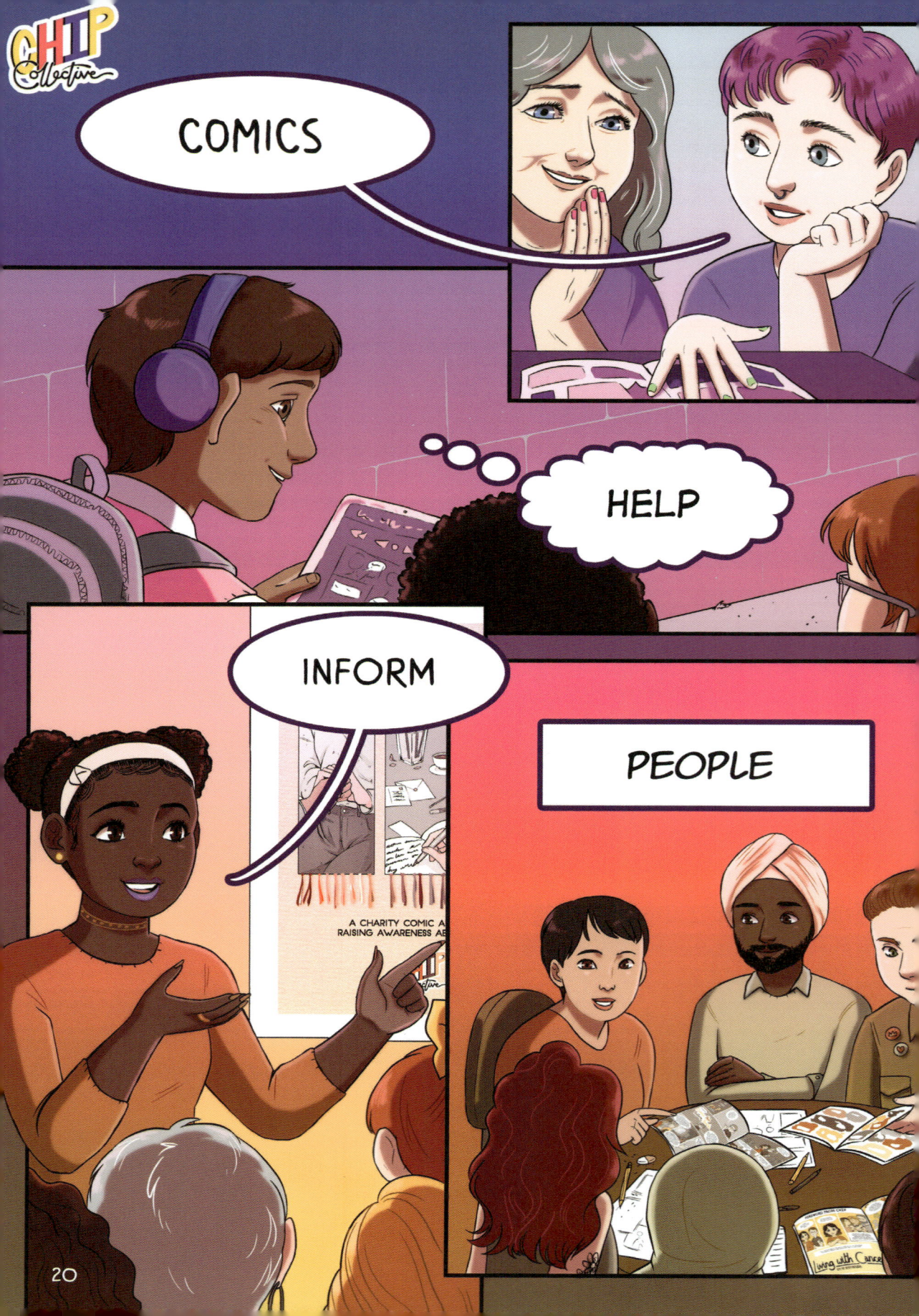

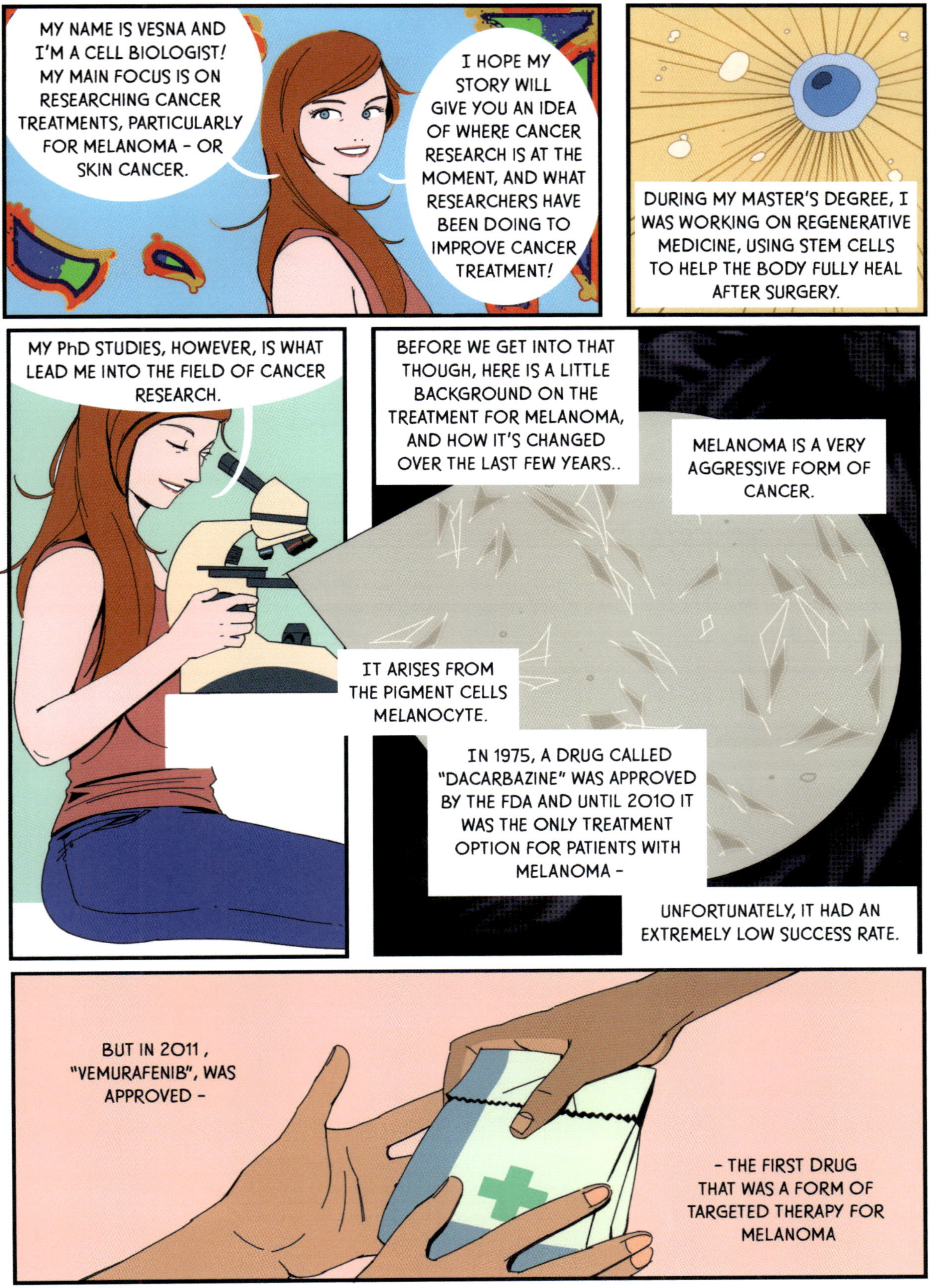

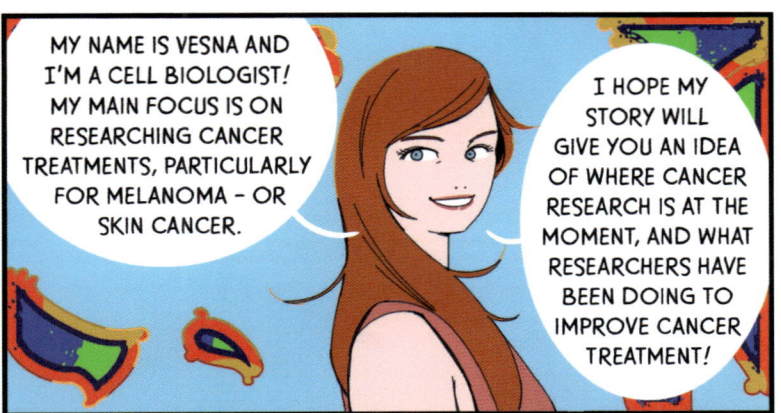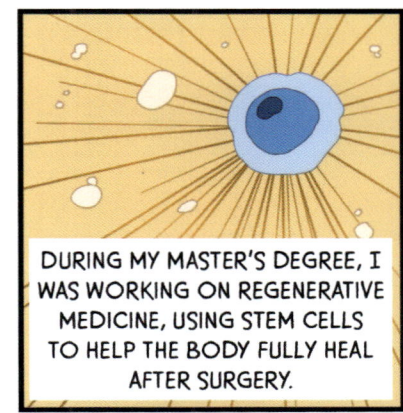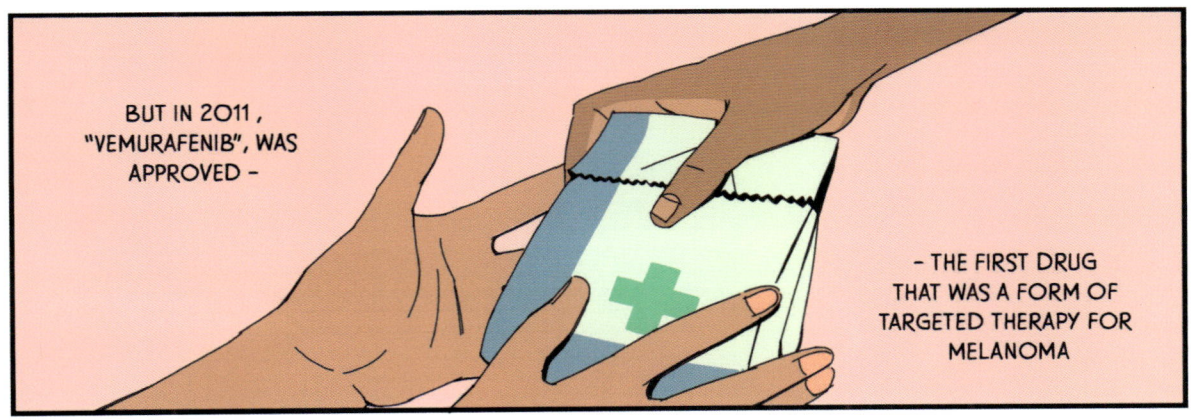

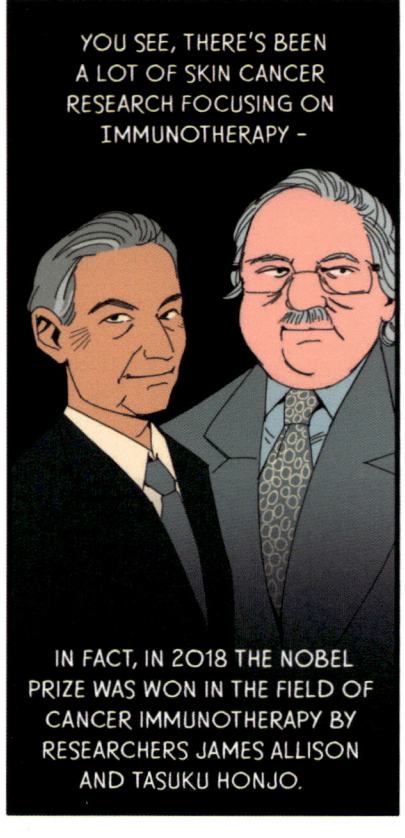
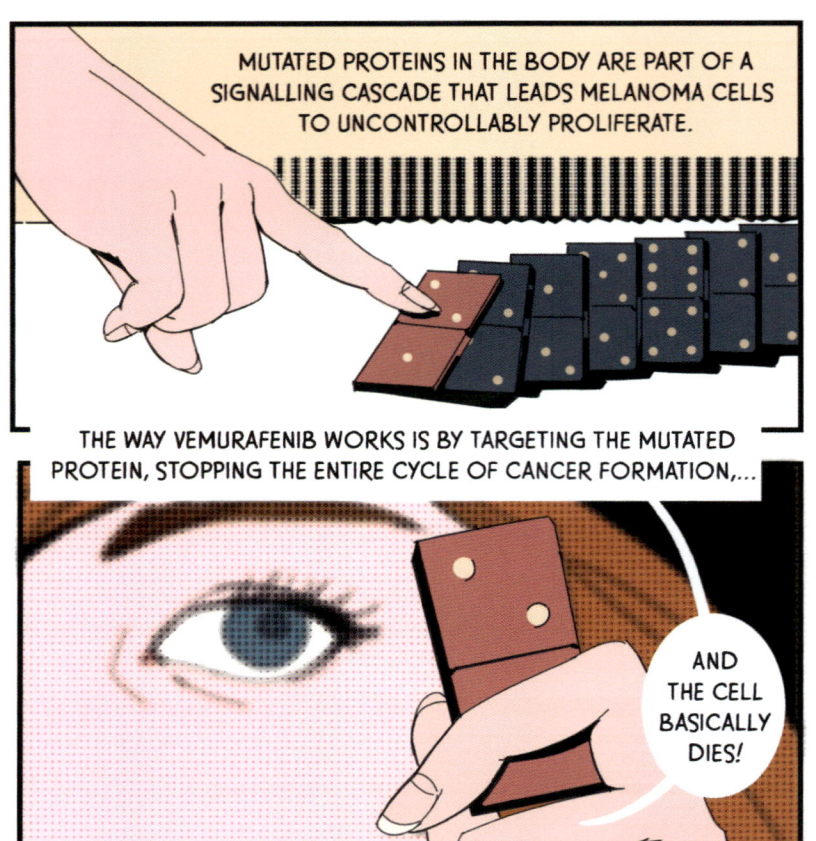
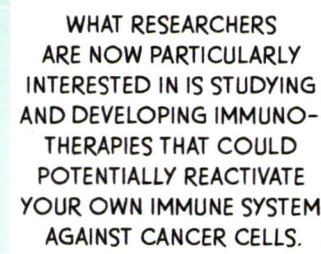
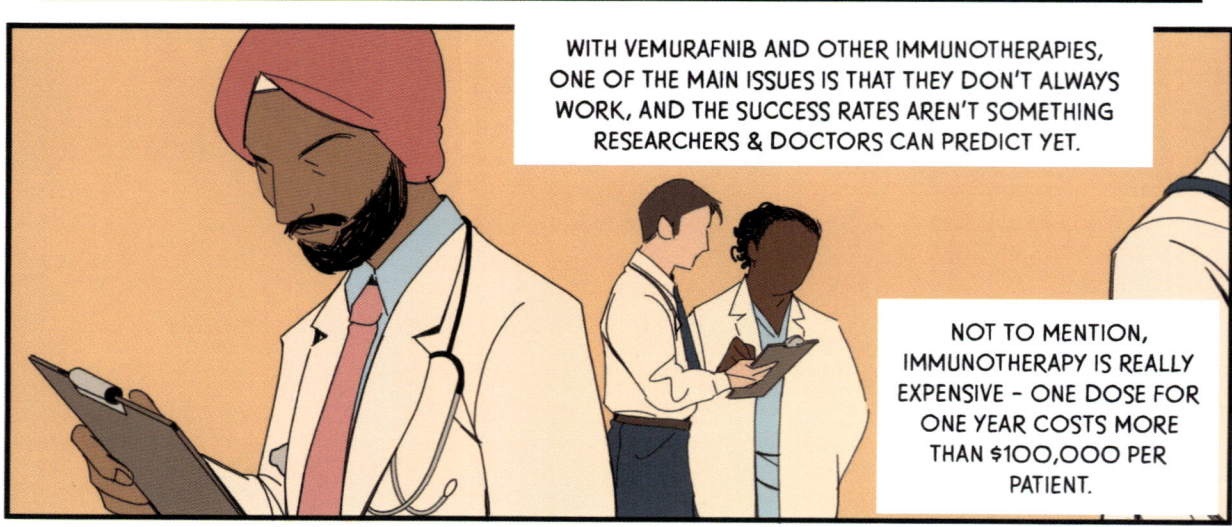

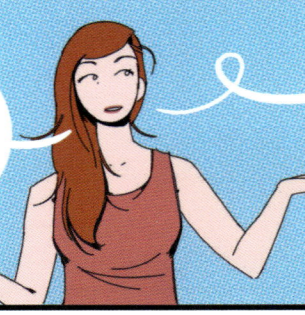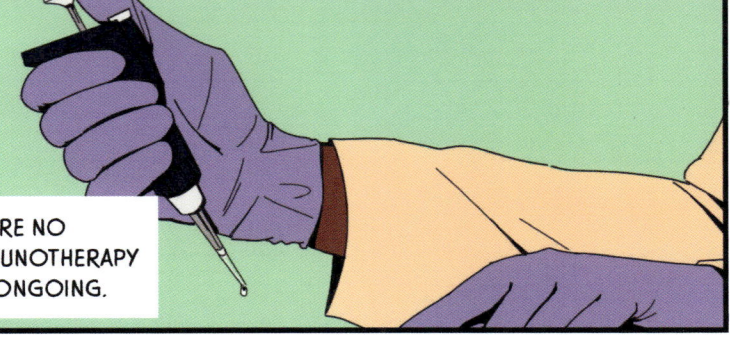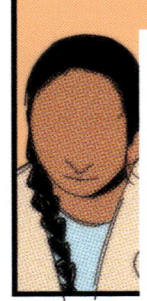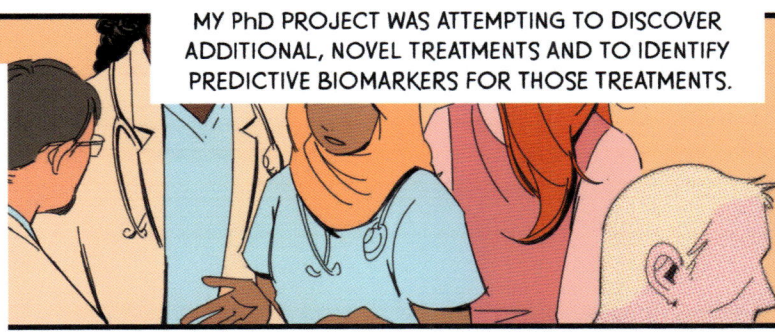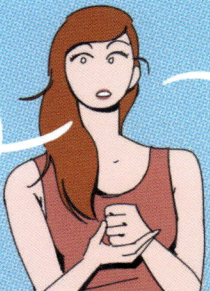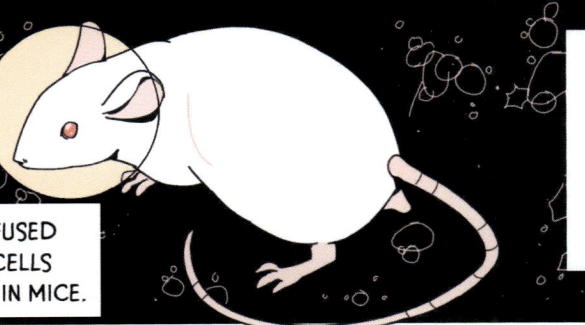

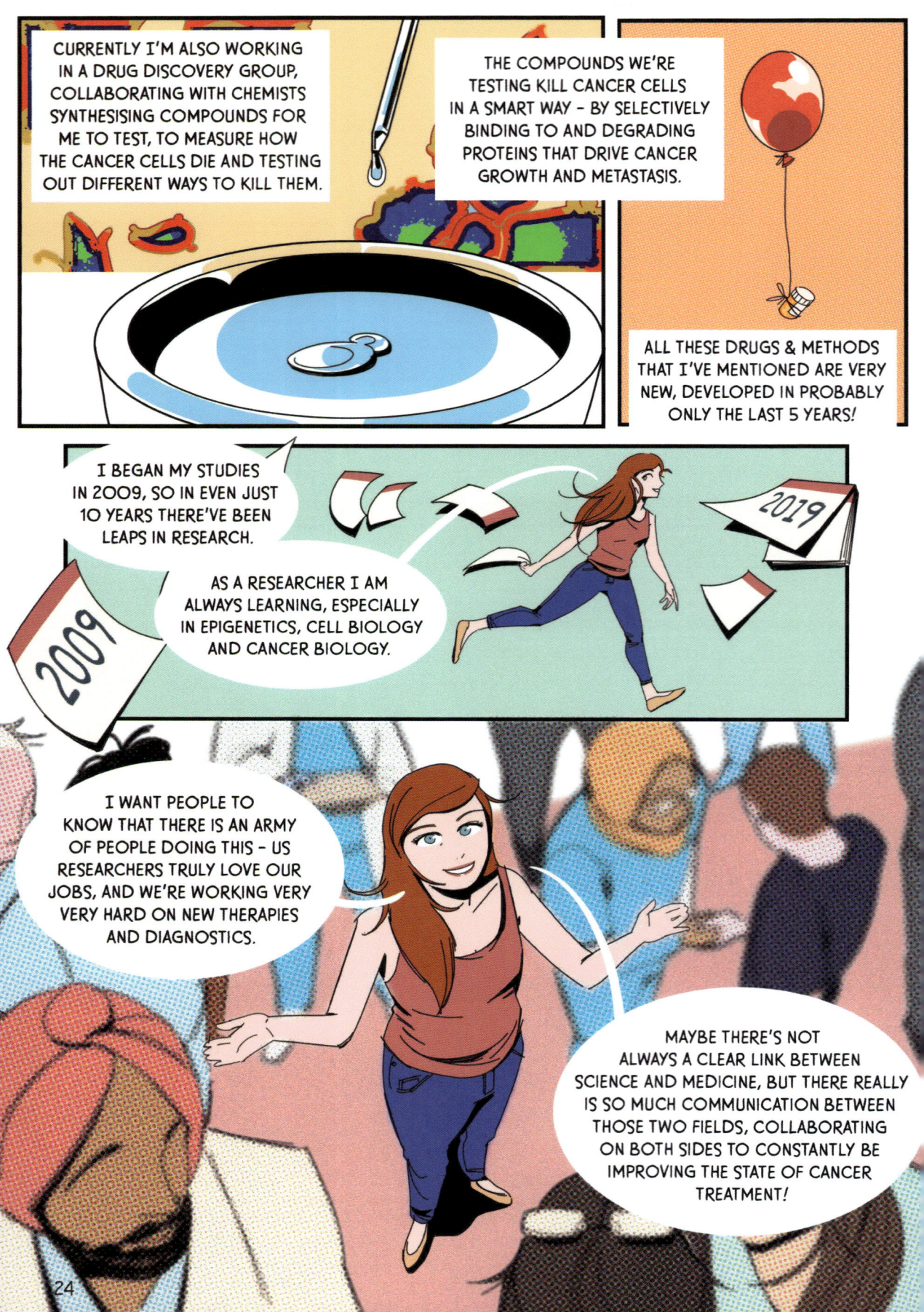

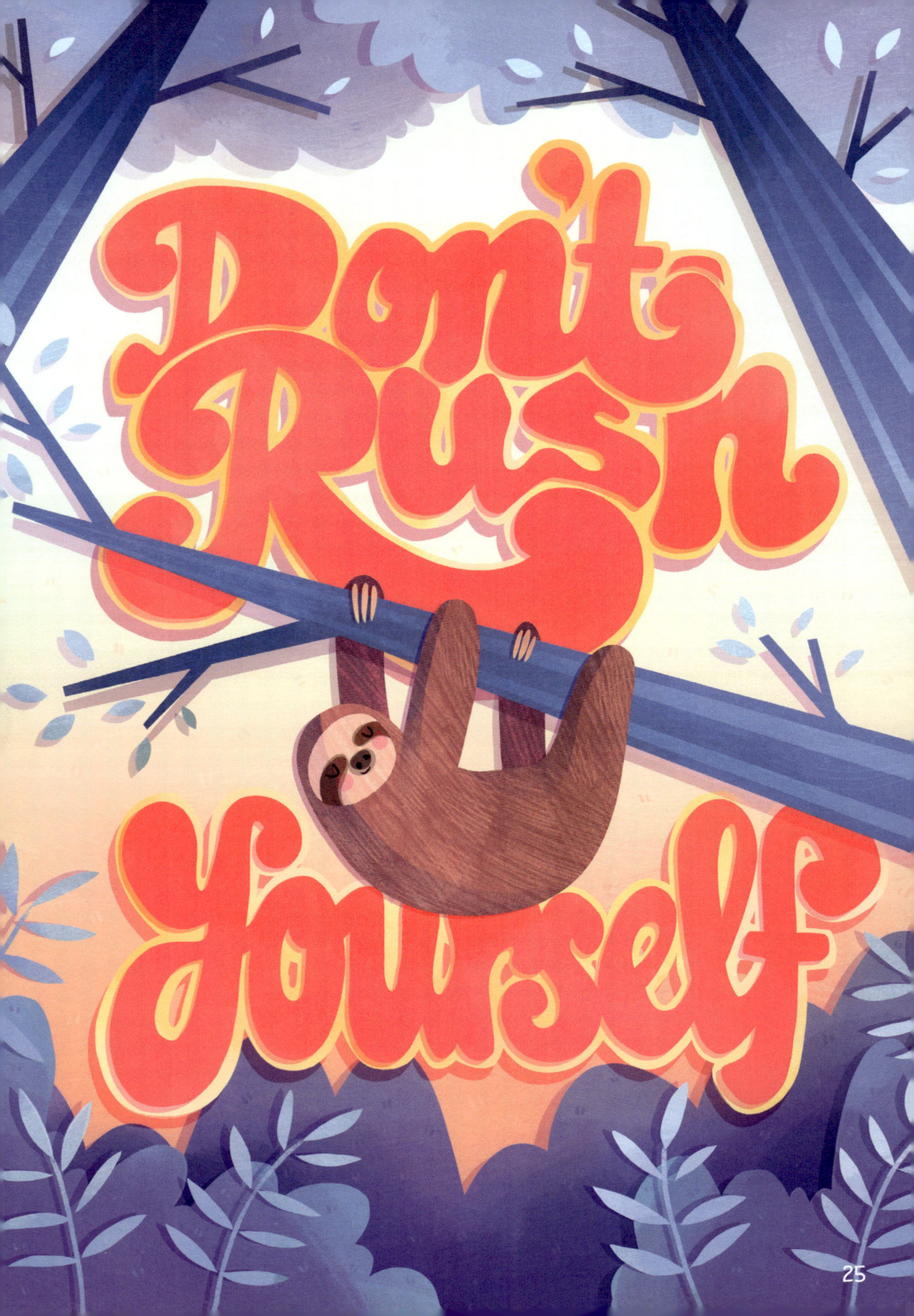

STAYING POSITIVE, KEEPING TOGETHER

STORY - RAJ | ART AND SCRIPT - CATRIONA LAIRD

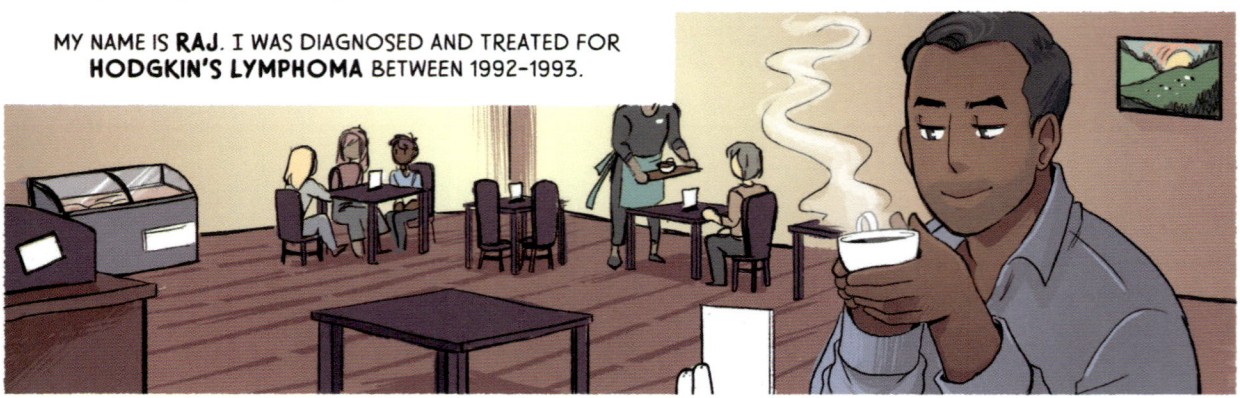

MY NAME IS **RAJ**. I WAS DIAGNOSED AND TREATED FOR **HODGKIN'S LYMPHOMA** BETWEEN 1992–1993.

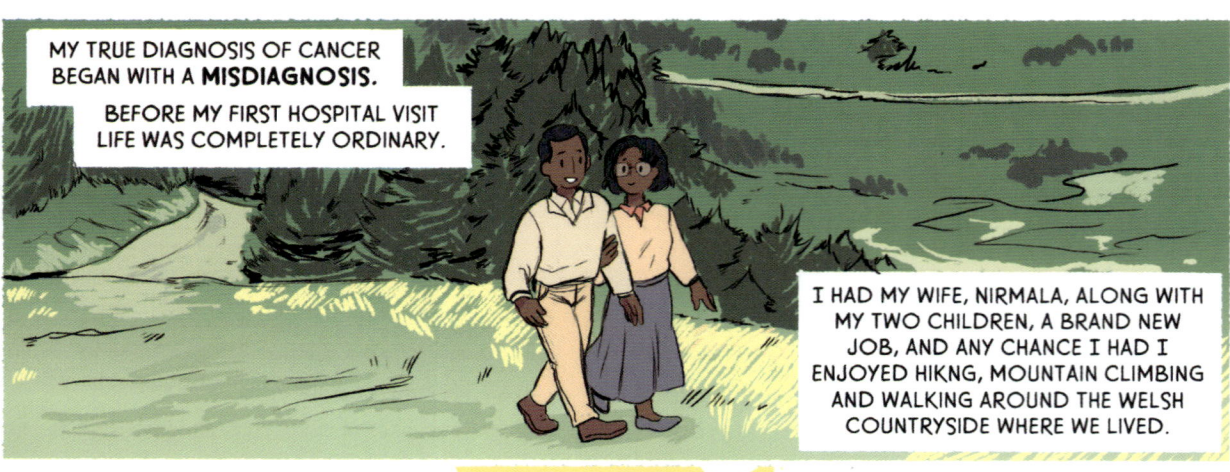

MY TRUE DIAGNOSIS OF CANCER BEGAN WITH A **MISDIAGNOSIS**.

BEFORE MY FIRST HOSPITAL VISIT LIFE WAS COMPLETELY ORDINARY.

I HAD MY WIFE, NIRMALA, ALONG WITH MY TWO CHILDREN, A BRAND NEW JOB, AND ANY CHANCE I HAD I ENJOYED HIKNG, MOUNTAIN CLIMBING AND WALKING AROUND THE WELSH COUNTRYSIDE WHERE WE LIVED.

I WAS VERY ACTIVE AND HEALTHY UNTIL ONE PARTICULAR WALK...

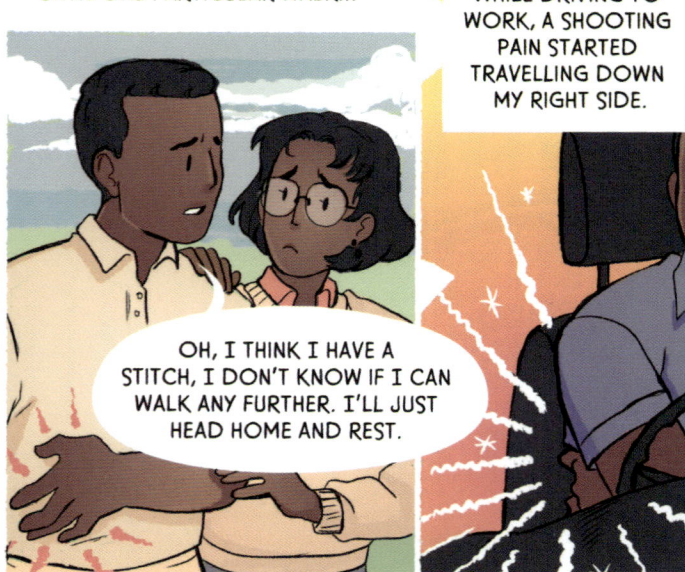

"OH, I THINK I HAVE A STITCH, I DON'T KNOW IF I CAN WALK ANY FURTHER. I'LL JUST HEAD HOME AND REST."

SOON AFTER THAT, WHILE DRIVING TO WORK, A SHOOTING PAIN STARTED TRAVELLING DOWN MY RIGHT SIDE.

I CALLED MY DOCTOR AND WAS ADMITTED TO HOSPITAL. I WAS DISCHARGED AFTER A FEW DAYS WHEN NO CAUSE OF THE PAIN WAS FOUND. WHEN THE PAIN RETURNED I WAS DIAGNOSED WITH **GRUMBLING APPENDICITIS** WHERE THE APPENDIX IS THREATENING TO RUPTURE BUT ISN'T URGENTLY NEEDING REMOVAL.

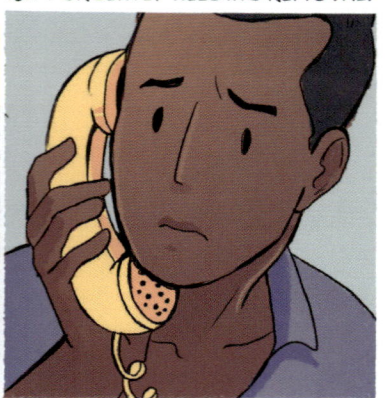

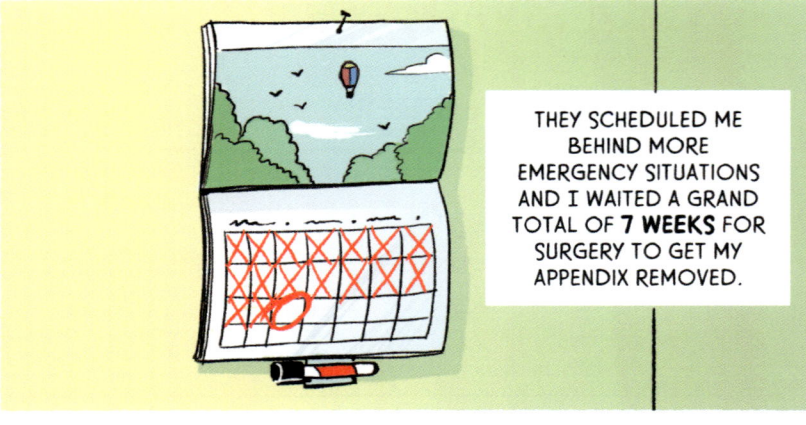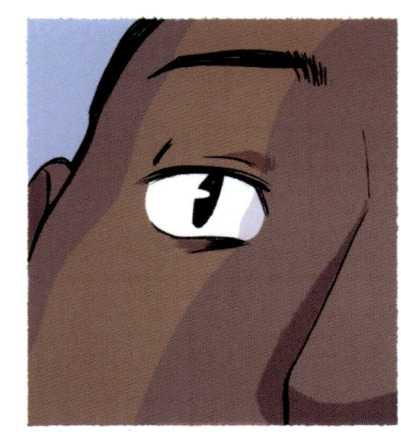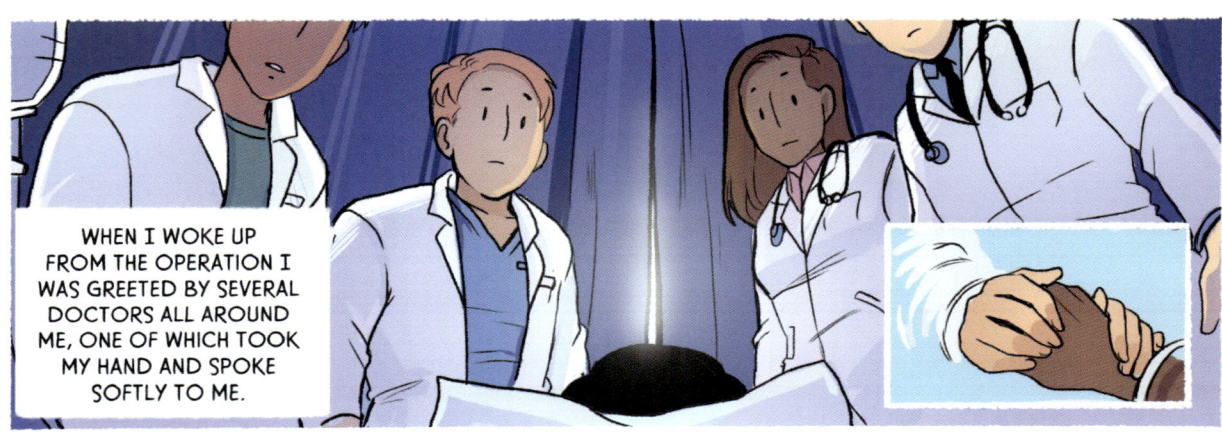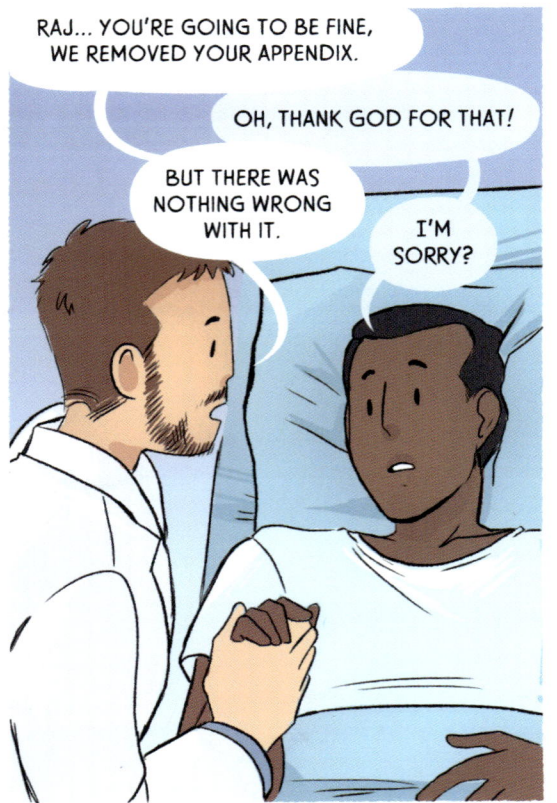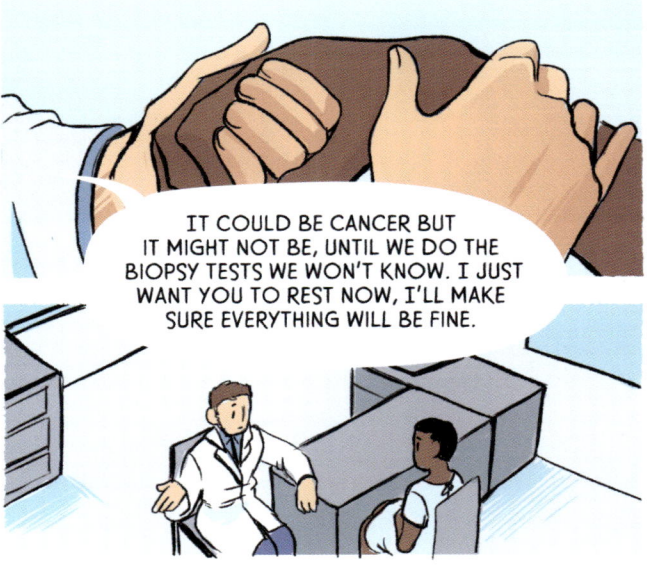

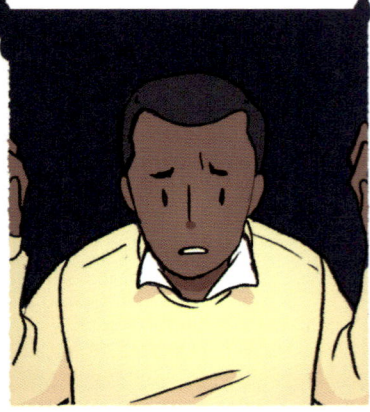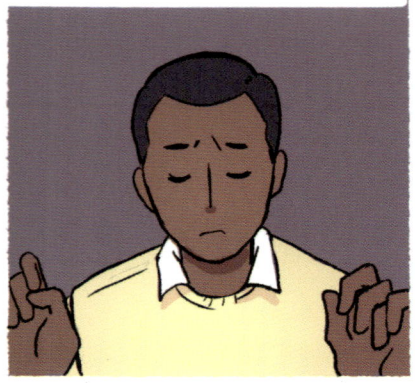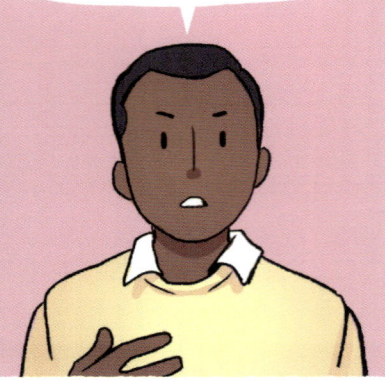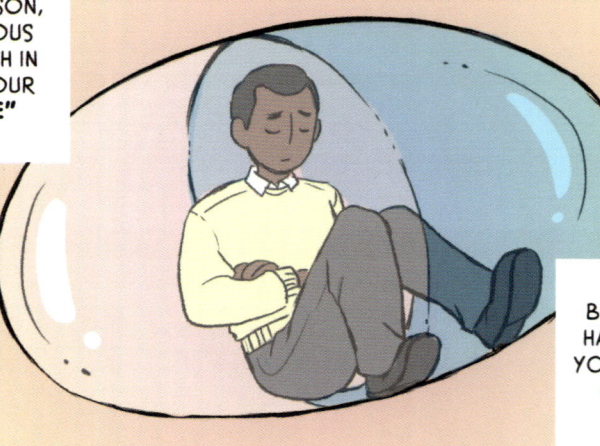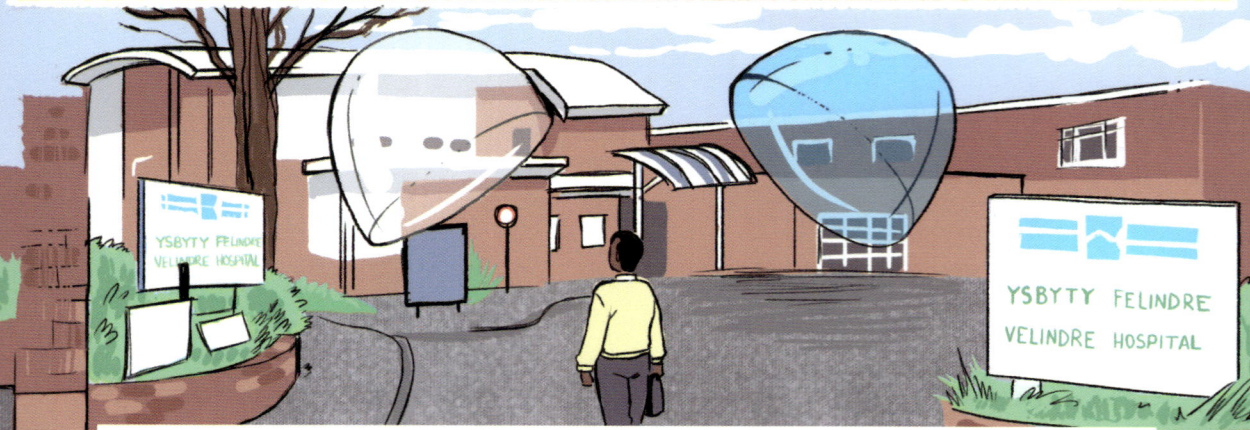

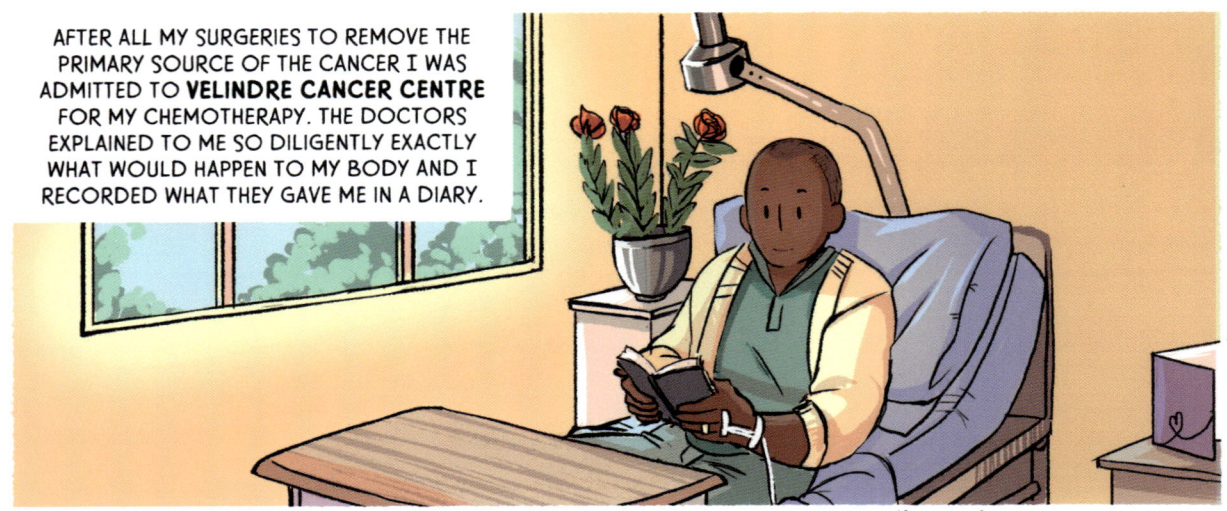

AFTER ALL MY SURGERIES TO REMOVE THE PRIMARY SOURCE OF THE CANCER I WAS ADMITTED TO **VELINDRE CANCER CENTRE** FOR MY CHEMOTHERAPY. THE DOCTORS EXPLAINED TO ME SO DILIGENTLY EXACTLY WHAT WOULD HAPPEN TO MY BODY AND I RECORDED WHAT THEY GAVE ME IN A DIARY.

IT WAS HUGELY COMFORTING TO RECEIVE CARDS FROM PEOPLE THINKING OF ME. MY WIFE, FAMILY AND FRIENDS ALSO PRAYED FOR MY WELLBEING.

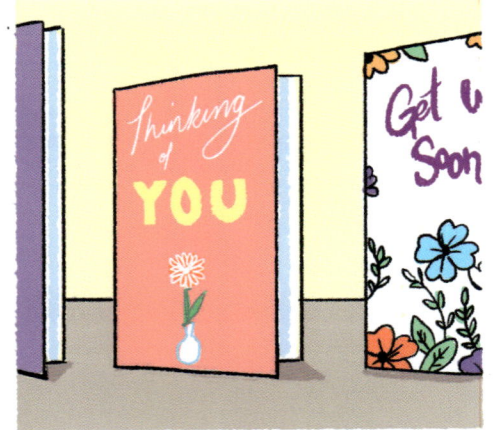

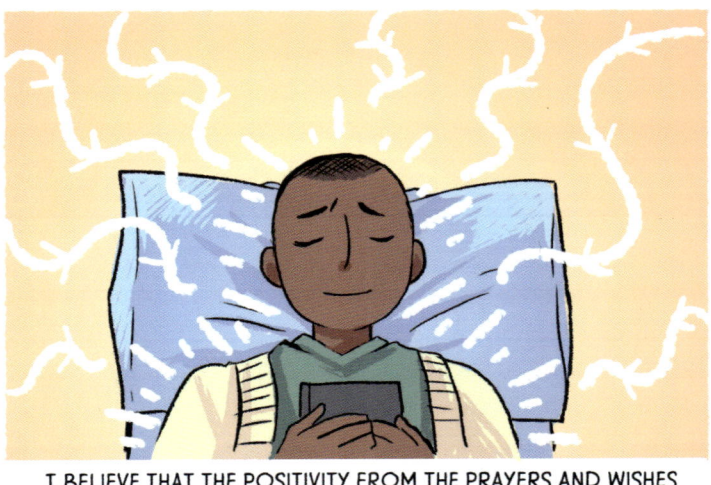

I BELIEVE THAT THE POSITIVITY FROM THE PRAYERS AND WISHES CAME TOGETHER, LIKE A TELEPHONE LINE, AND REACHED ME. THE POSITIVENESS OF THAT CHARGE CAME INTO MY SYSTEM AND **KEPT ME FIGHTING ON.**

BY THE END OF MY LONG AND DIFFICULT TREATMENT THEY DECLARED ME CANCER FREE – **THE COURSE HAD BEEN A SUCCESS.**

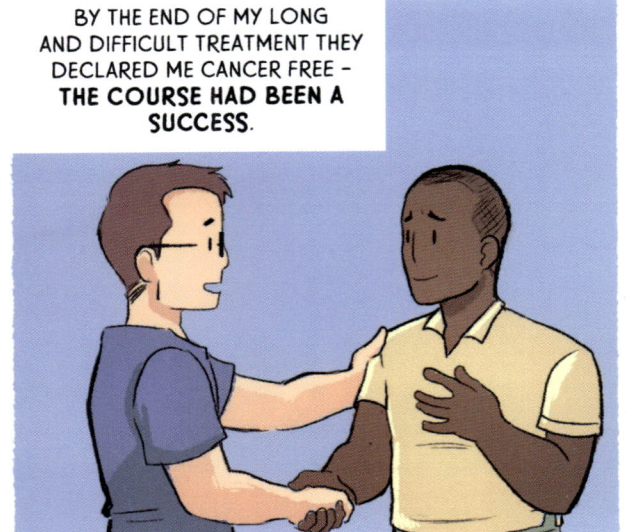

LIFE WAS VERY DIFFERENT THOUGH, I HAD TO REALLY THINK ABOUT **WHAT I WANTED TO DO WITH MYSELF.**

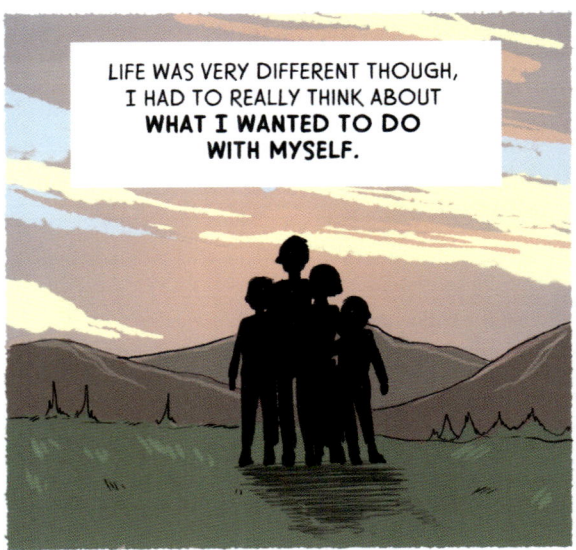

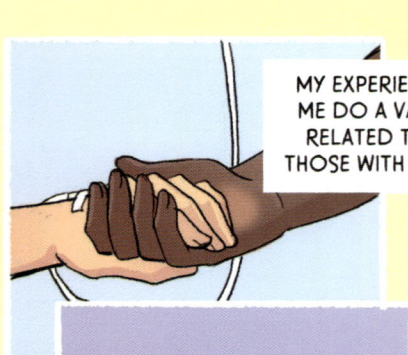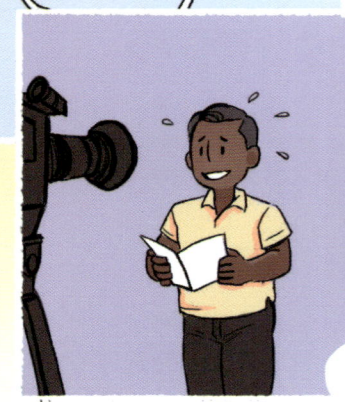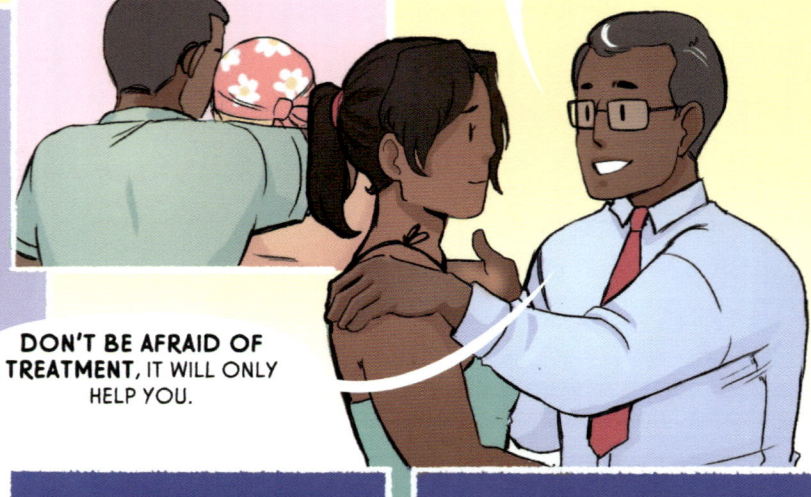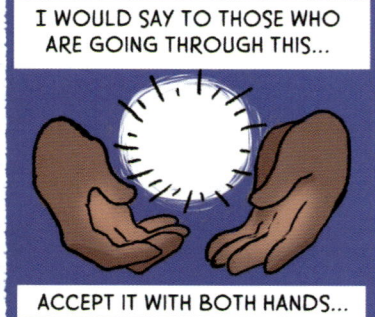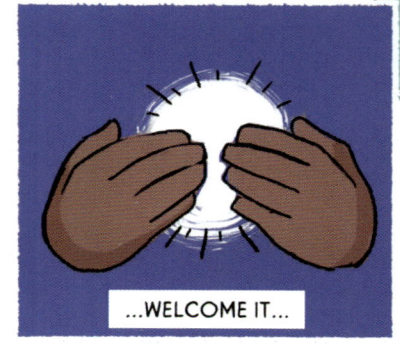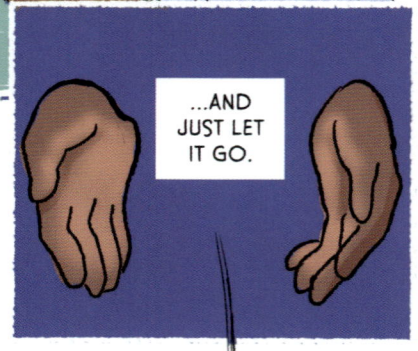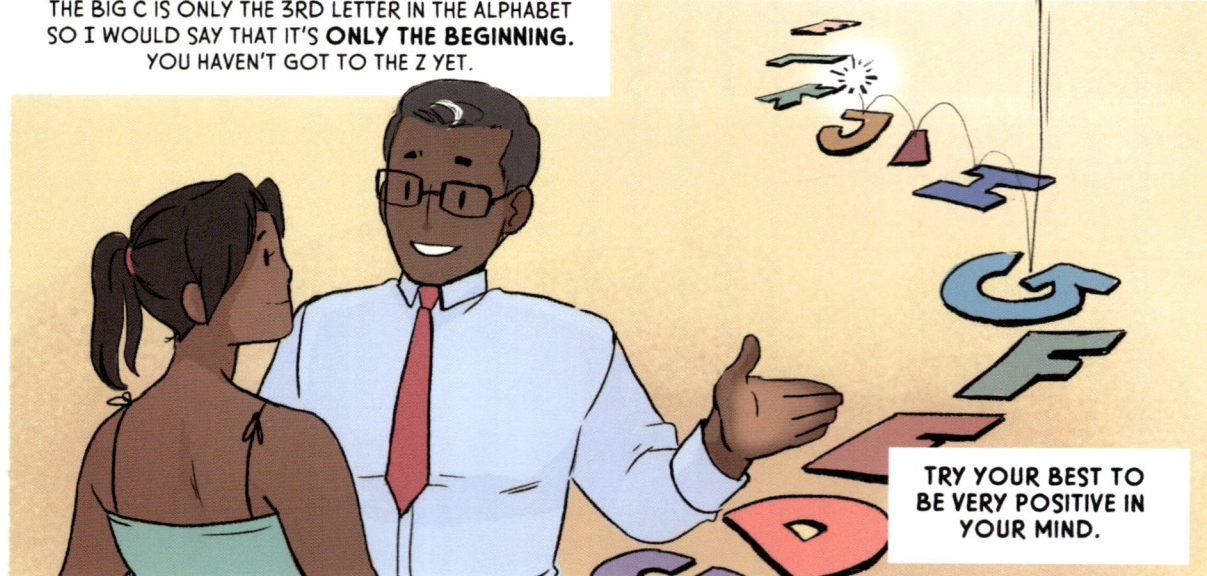

"accept it welcome it and let it go"

mairi Isla 2019

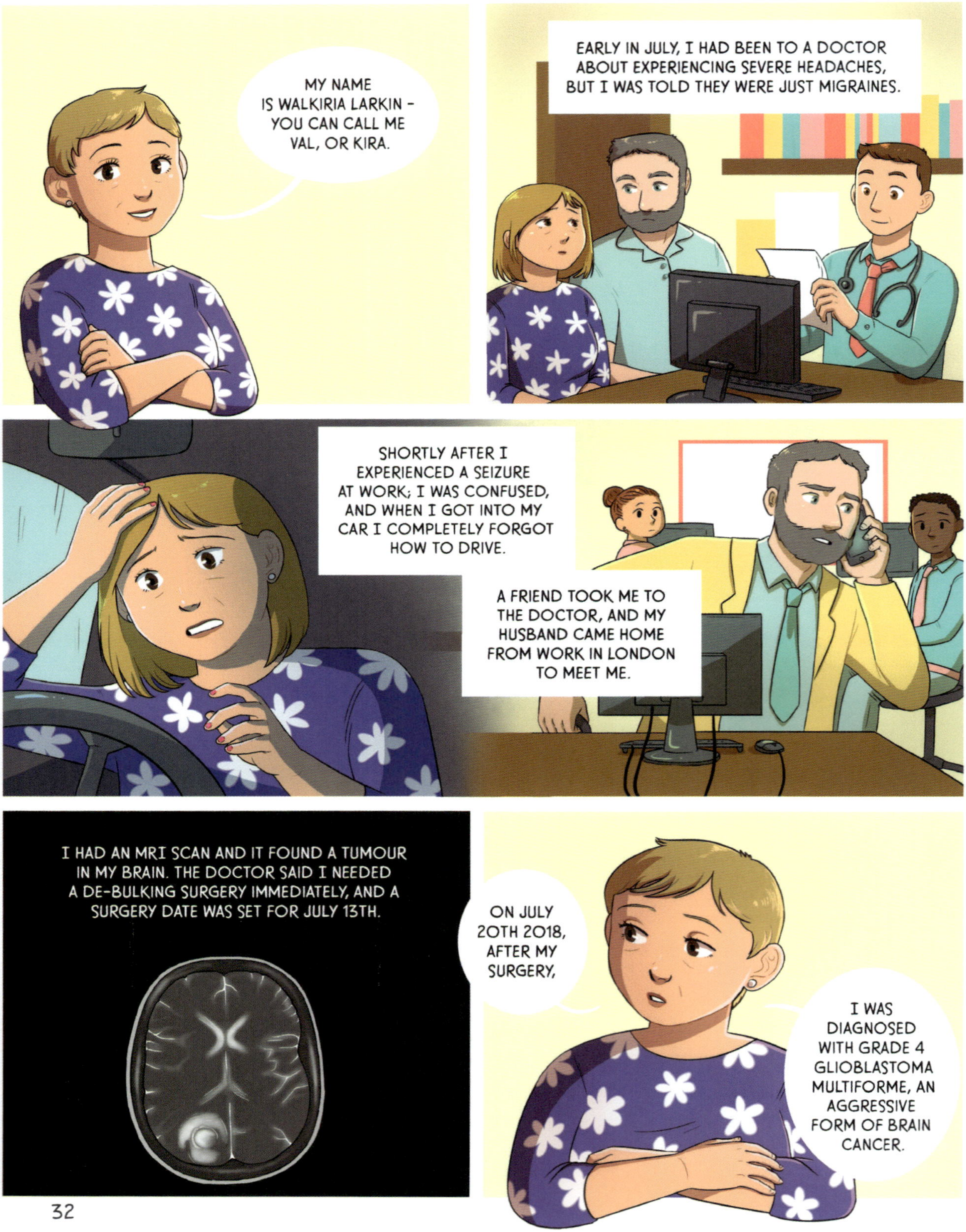

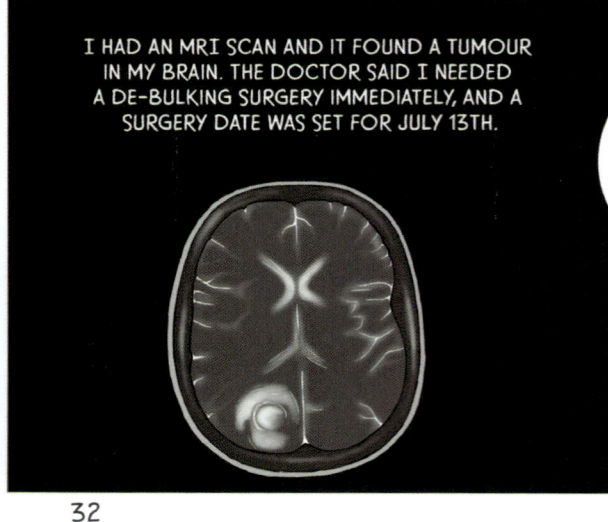
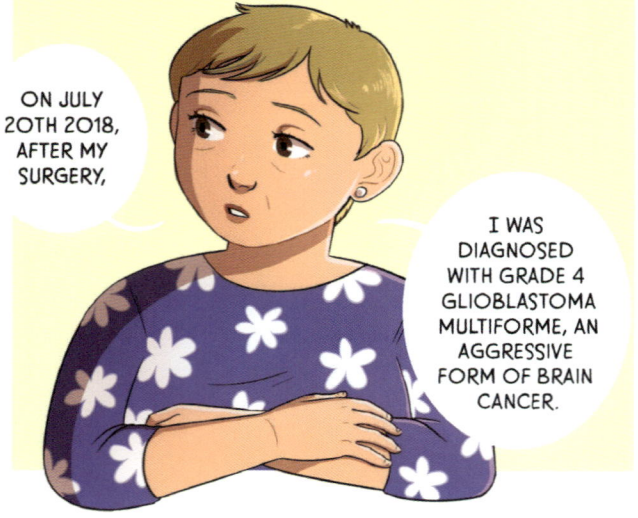

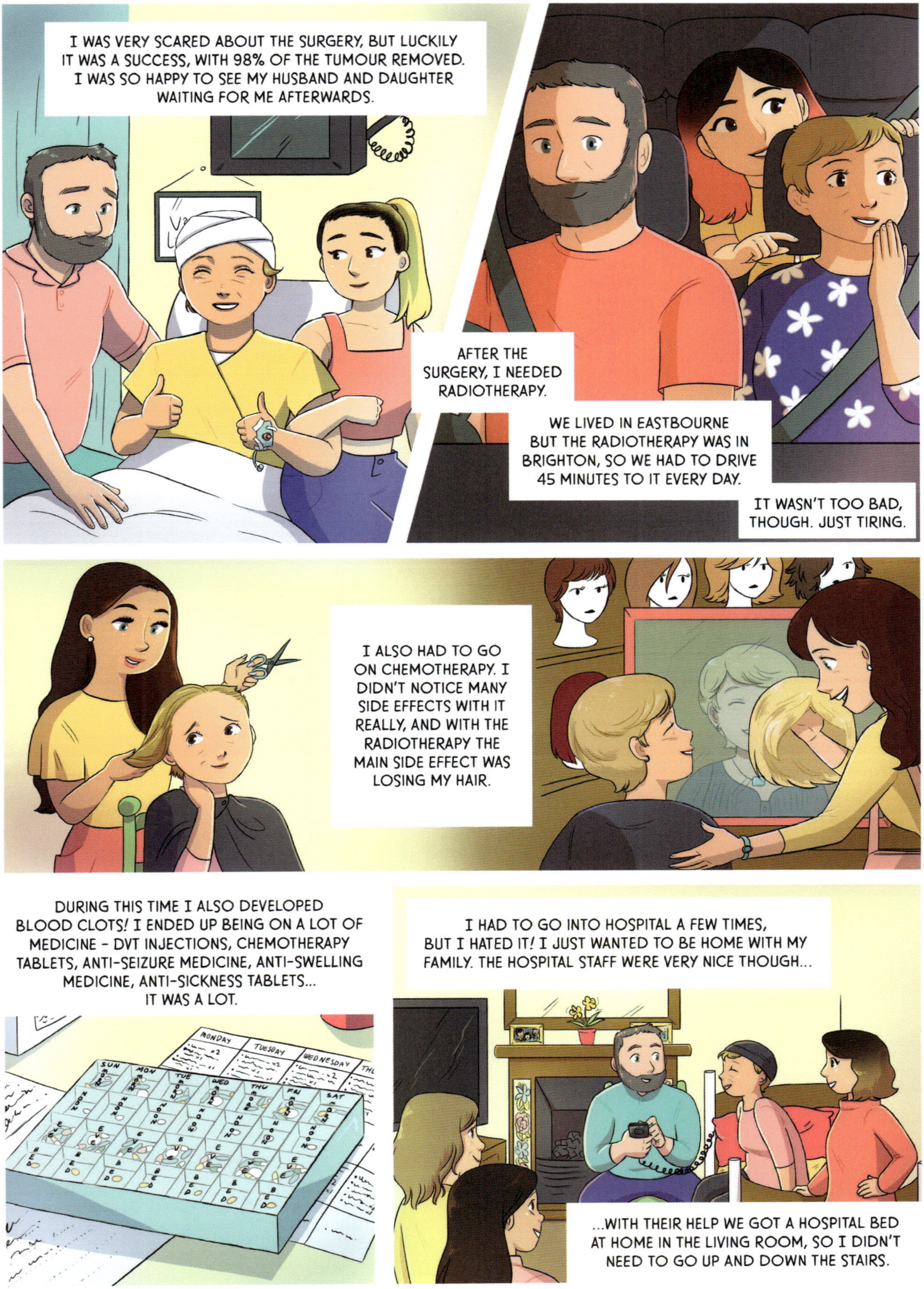

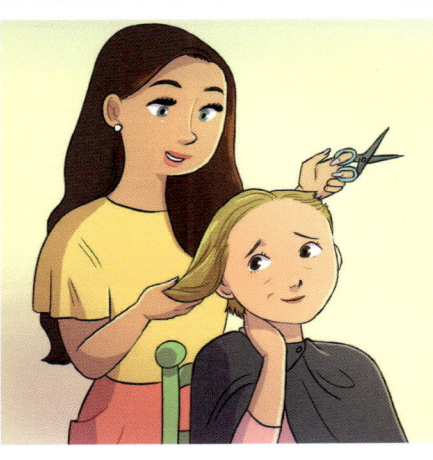
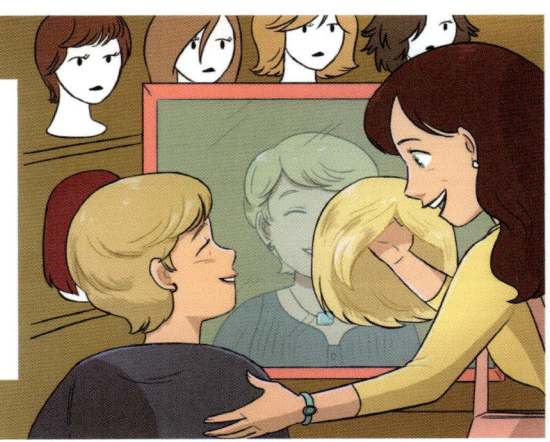
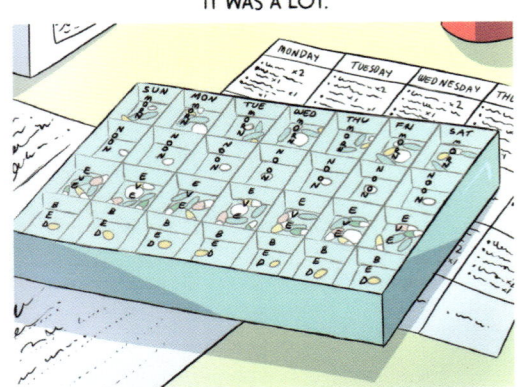
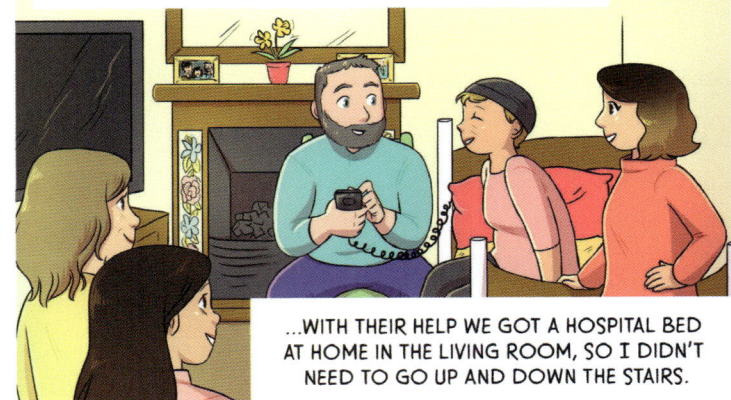

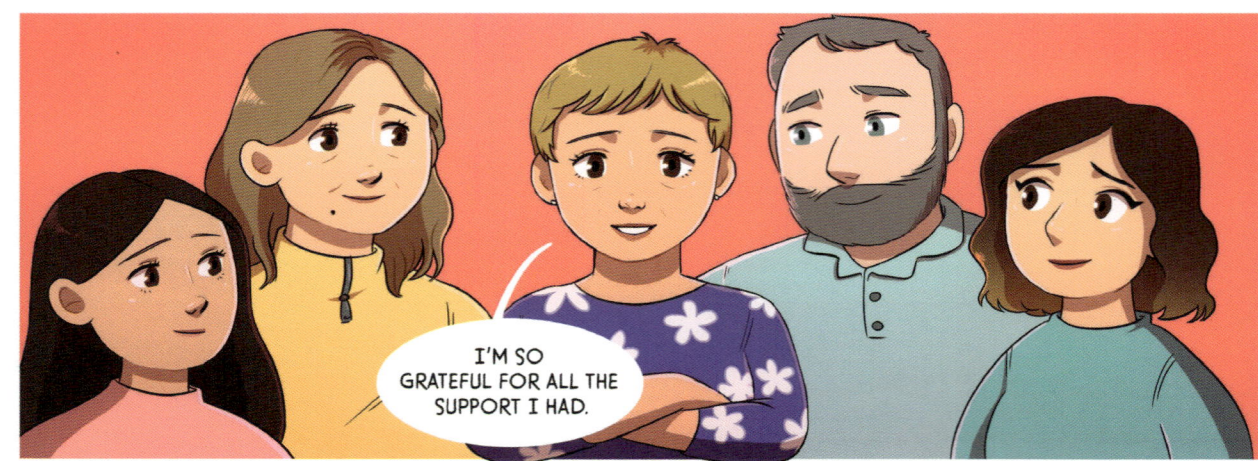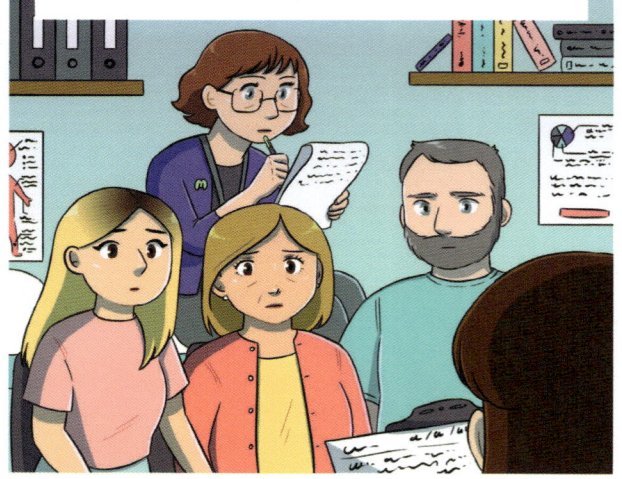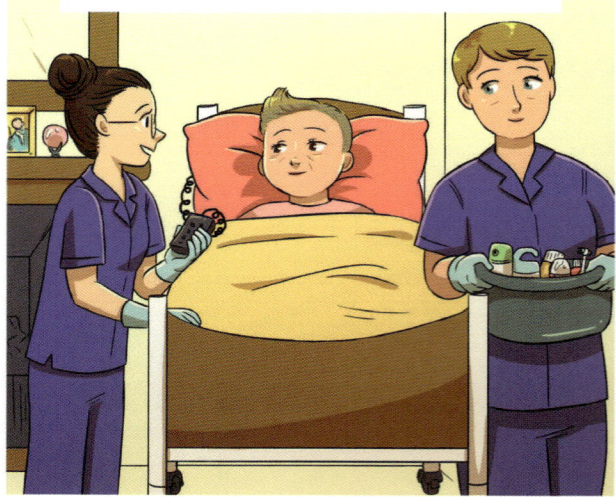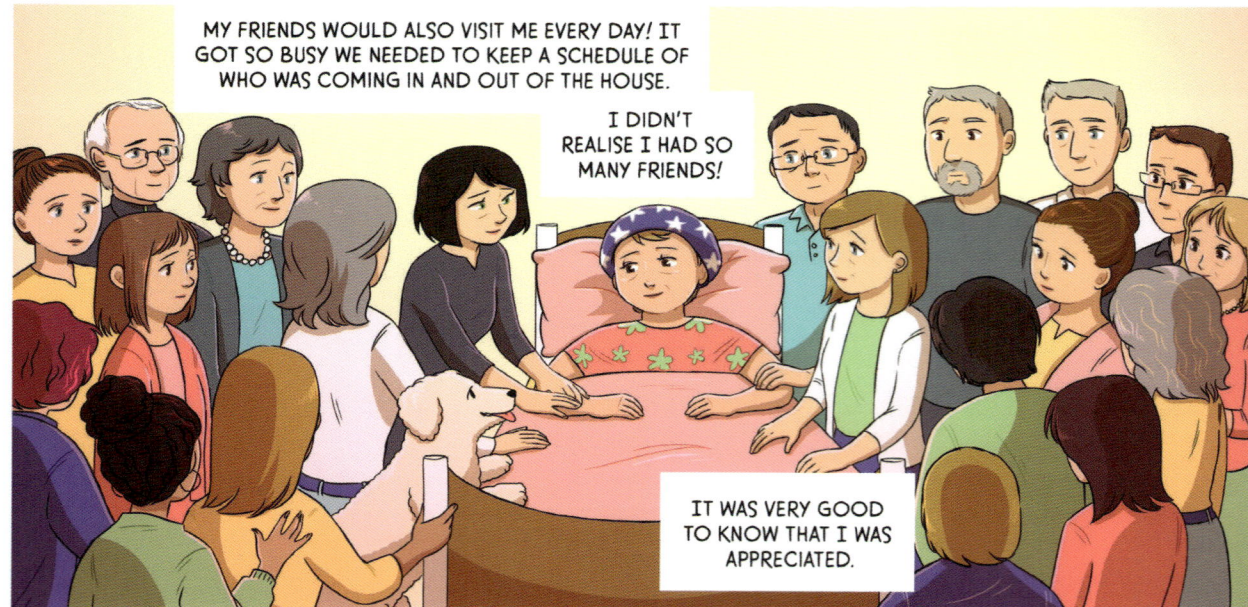

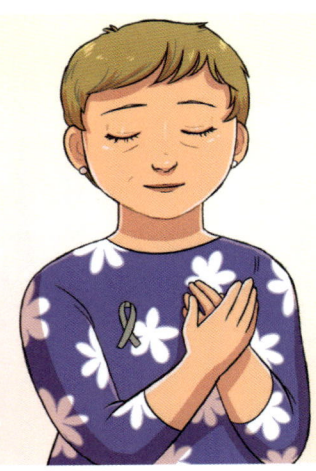

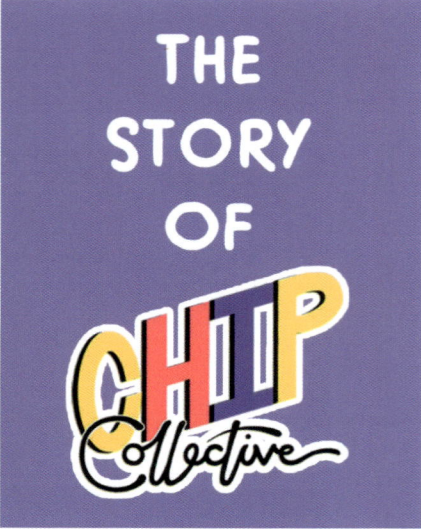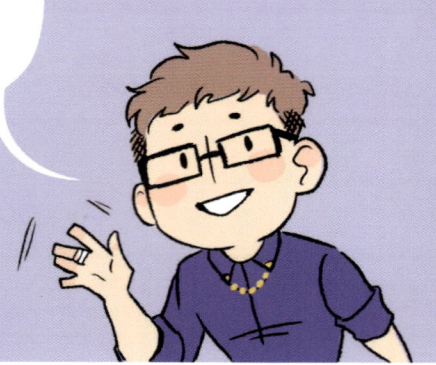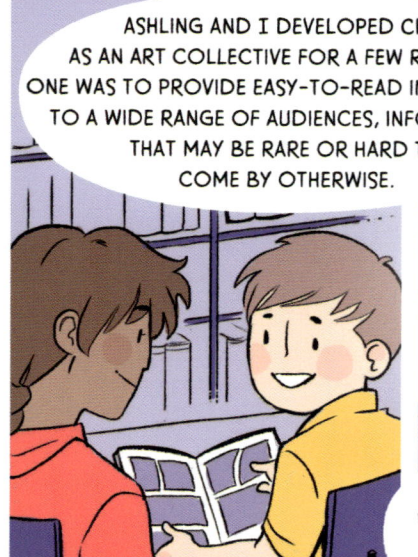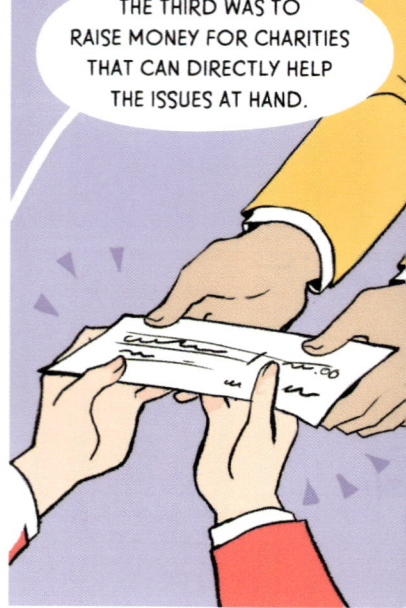

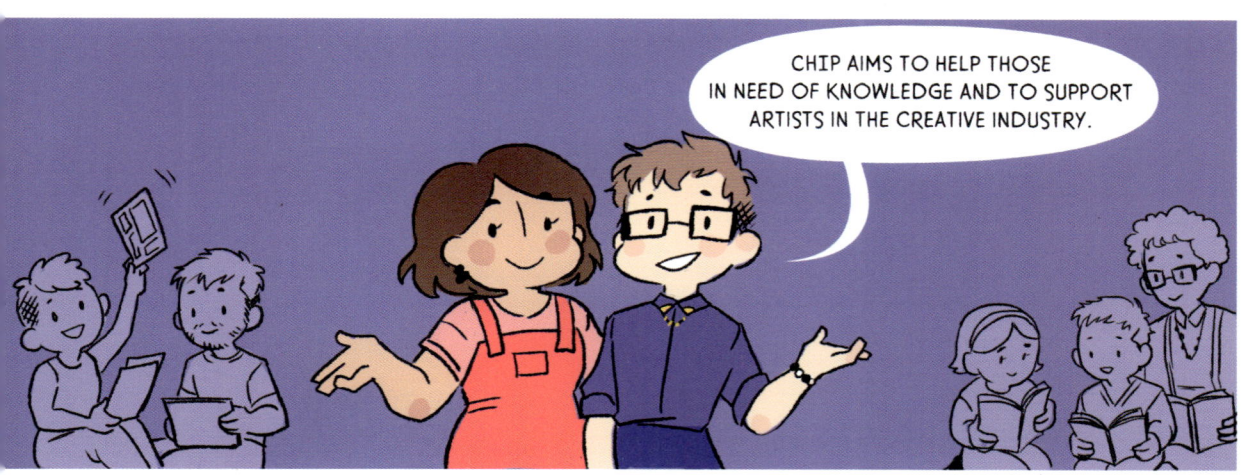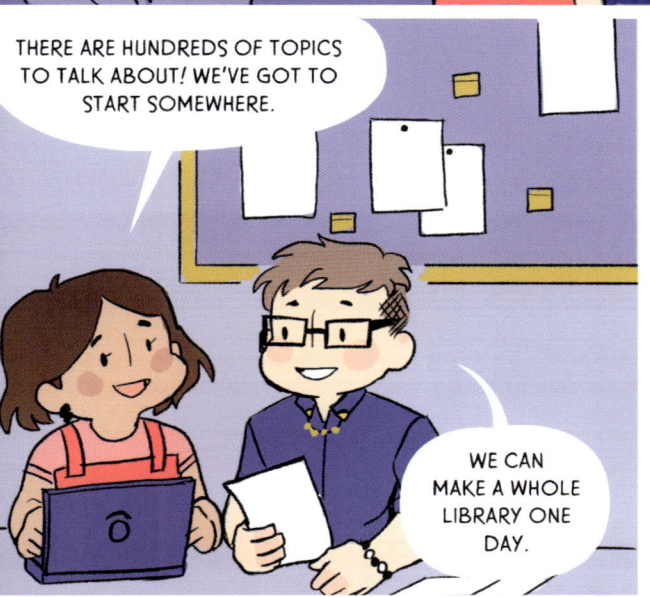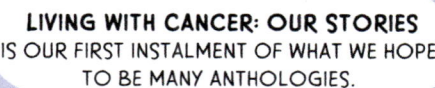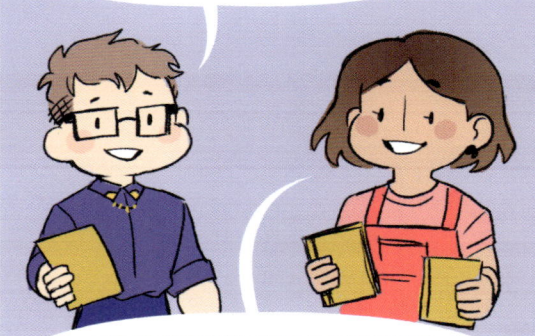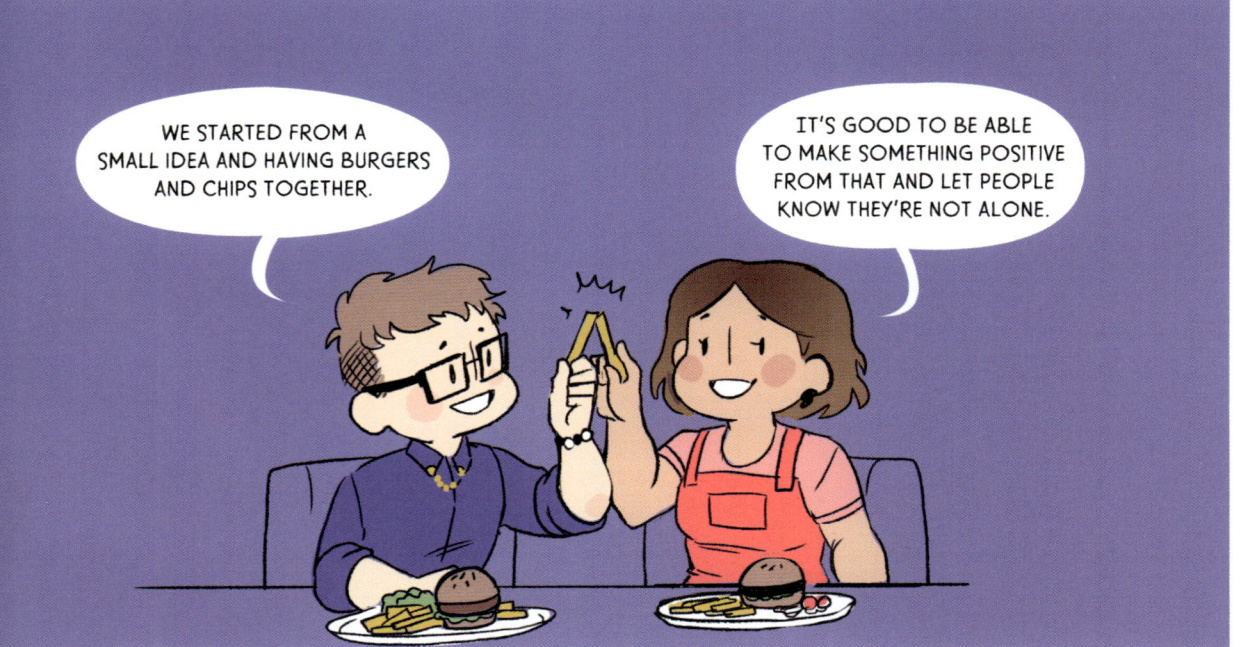

CONTRIBUTORS

CREATING A COMIC ANTHOLOGY REQUIRES THE TIME, EFFORT AND SKILLS OF MANY PEOPLE IN ORDER TO BECOME A REALITY.
LIVING WITH CANCER: OUR STORIES HAS BEEN MADE WITH THE HELP OF THE FOLLOWING PEOPLE.

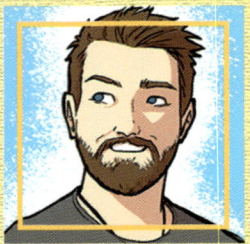

ELLIOT BALSON ILLUSTRATED ANN'S STORY (PAGES 15-19)
ELLIOT IS A COMIC ARTIST, LETTERER AND ILLUSTRATOR. HE BELIEVES CHIP IS AN EXCELLENT OPPORTUNITY FOR PEOPLE TO HAVE THEIR STORIES AND VOICES HEARD; CREATED IN A SUPPORTIVE AND DIRECT WAY. ARTISTS WANT THEIR WORK TO MEAN SOMETHING TO PEOPLE AND CHIP IS OUT TO DO JUST THAT.

WEBSITE: ARTSTATION.COM/ELLBALSON
TWITTER: @ELLBALSONART

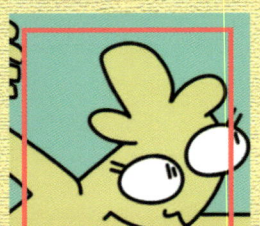

EVE GREENWOOD ILLUSTRATED CARLY'S STORY (PAGES 11-13)
EVE IS A COMIC ARTIST, WRITER AND ILLUSTRATOR. THEY BELIEVE COMICS ARE A WONDERFUL MEDIUM THROUGH WHICH TO SHARE THE STORIES AND VOICES OF THOSE WHO WILL OTHERWISE GO UNHEARD OF. THEY ARE EXCITED TO BE PART OF SUCH AN IMPORTANT PROJECT.

WEBSITE: EVEGWOOD.COM
TWITTER: @EVEGWOOD

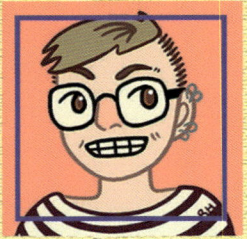

REBECCA HORNER ILLUSTRATED THE POSTER ON PAGE 4
REBECCA IS A CARTOONIST AND COLOURIST. WITH A MASTER'S IN COMICS, REBECCA CONSIDERS HERSELF A JACK OF VARIOUS TRADES. SHE WANTED TO GET INVOLVED WITH THIS PROJECT BECAUSE CANCER IS A TOPIC THAT HITS TOO CLOSE TO HOME FOR MANY OF US, AND IT'S IMPORTANT TO SHARE THOSE STORIES.

WEBSITE: REBECCAHORNER.COM
TWITTER: @REEKUS

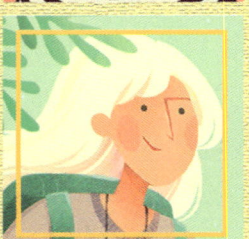

SARAH HOLLIDAY ILLUSTRATED THE POSTER ON PAGE 25
SARAH IS AN ILLUSTRATOR WHO ENJOYS CREATING COLOURFUL, STYLISED ILLUSTRATIONS, OFTEN INSPIRED BY NATURE AND TRANQUILITY. SHE'S PROUD TO BE CONTRIBUTING TO SUCH AN IMPORTANT PROJECT AND HOPES THAT HER ART CAN HELP MAKE THE WORLD A TINY BIT BRIGHTER.

WEBSITE: SARAHHOLLIDAYART.COM
TWITTER: @SARAHHOLIDAY

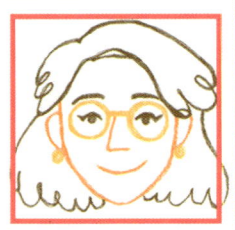

MAIRI ISLA ILLUSTRATED THE POSTER ON PAGE 31
MAIRI IS AN ILLUSTRATOR, MAKER AND SHINY SHOE ENTHUSIAST. MAIRI LIKES TO DABBLE IN ALL SORTS OF PROCESSES - INCLUDING CERAMICS AND PRINT-MAKING AS WELL AS TRADITIONAL METHODS. SHE FEELS PRIVILEGED TO HELP PEOPLE SHARE THEIR PERSONAL EXPERIENCES WITH OTHERS AND HOPEFULLY SPREAD POSITIVITY THROUGH THEIR STORIES.

WEBSITE: MAIRI-ISLA.COM
TWITTER: @MAIRI_ISLA

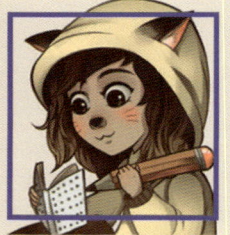

SARA JULIA ILLUSTRATED NAOMI'S STORY (PAGES 5 TO 9)
SARA IS AN ILLUSTRATOR, COMIC ARTIST AND WRITER. SARA HAS BEEN READING AND DRAWING COMICS FOR AS LONG AS SHE CAN REMEMBER. COMICS HAVE HELPED HER GET THROUGH SOME TOUGH TIMES! SHE HOPES TO DO JUSTICE TO THE STORIES IN THIS PROJECT.

WEBSITE: SARALJART.COM
TWITTER: @SWISSCHOCOLATEART

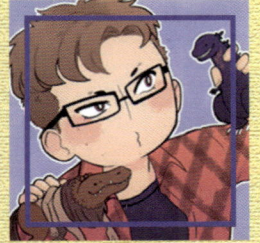

CATRIONA LAIRD ILLUSTRATED RAJ'S STORY (PAGES 26-30) AND THE POSTER ON PAGE 10

CATRIONA IS AN ARTIST, DESIGNER AND ONE OF CHIP'S CO-FOUNDERS. THEY HELPED CREATE CHIP COLLECTIVE BECAUSE THERE ARE PEOPLE WHO NEED THEIR STORIES TOLD BUT DON'T HAVE THE VOICES TO SAY IT. THEY WANT TO GIVE THEM THAT VOICE THROUGH ARTWORK AND TELL THEIR TALES.

WEBSITE: CATRIONALAIRD.CO.UK
TWITTER: @OWLROOSTART

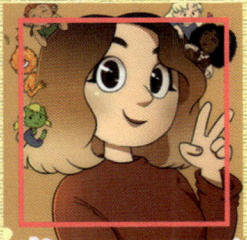

ASHLING LARKIN ILLUSTRATED WALKIRIA'S STORY (PAGES 32-35) AND THE POSTERS ON PAGES 14 AND 20

ASHLING IS AN ARTIST AND ONE OF CHIP'S CO-FOUNDERS, PROJECT MANAGER AND SOCIAL MEDIA MANAGER. ASHLING HELPED CREATE CHIP BECAUSE SHE BELIEVES IN THE ABILITY OF COMICS ASSISTING PEOPLE BOTH IN HEART AND MIND. SHE'S PROUD OF WHAT WE'RE DOING AND EXCITED TO SEE OUR UPCOMING PROJECTS BECOME A REALITY THAT MAY POSITIVELY AFFECT PEOPLE'S LIVES.

WEBSITE: ASHLINGDRAWS.COM
TWITTER: @ASHLINGDRAWS

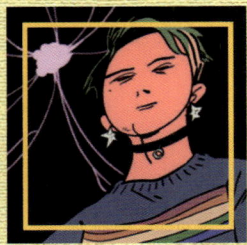

JULES VALERA ILLUSTRATED VESNA'S STORY (PAGES 21-24)

JULES IS A COMIC ARTIST AND ILLUSTRATOR. JULES DECIDED TO WORK WITH CHIP BECAUSE THEY THINK IT'S FASCINATING TO VISUALISE COMPLEX AND IMPORTANT MEDICAL RESEARCH. THROUGH COMICS WE CAN MAKE THIS INFORMATION EASILY ACCESSIBLE TO SO MANY MORE PEOPLE.

WEBSITE: SNAILESQUE.COM
TWITTER: @SNAILESQUE

THE STORYTELLERS

ANN'S STORY INVOLVES CARING FOR HER MOTHER WHEN SHE WAS DIAGNOSED WITH OVARIAN CANCER WHEN ANN WAS A STUDENT. THE TRAUMA AFFECTED ANN FOR MANY YEARS AND SHE SPEAKS OF HOW SHE AND HER FAMILY HAVE LEARNED TO COPE SINCE THE EVENTS OF THE STORY.

CARLY IS A BAND 5 CHILDREN'S NURSE WHO CARES FOR CHILDREN WHO ARE ADMITTED TO HOSPITAL FOR BONE MARROW TRANSPLANT TREATMENT. WHILE ONE ASPECT OF HER JOB IS LOOKING AFTER THE NEEDS OF THE KIDS, SHE DETAILS THE OTHER LESSER KNOWN PARTS OF HER JOB THAT SHE ALSO TAKES CARE OF.

NAOMI WAS DIAGNOSED WITH A FORM OF BRAIN CANCER AT ONLY 20 YEARS OLD. NAOMI TALKS ABOUT HOW MUCH CREATIVITY, WRITING AND ART HELPED HER THROUGH THIS DIFFICULT TIME IN HER LIFE AND HOW THE SUPPORT SHE RECEIVED CONTINUES TO HELP HER TO THIS DAY.

RAJ'S STORY CENTRES AROUND HIS SHEER POSITIVITY DURING HIS TREATMENT FOR HODGEKIN'S LYMPHOMA IN THE 90s AND HOW HIS FAMILY, FRIENDS AND COMMUNITY KEPT HIM STRONG ON HIS DARKEST DAYS. RAJ HAS USED HIS STORY TO HELP AND SUPPORT OTHERS GOING THROUGH SIMILAR SITUATIONS.

VESNA IS A CELL BIOLOGIST RESEARCHING EFFECTIVE TREATMENTS FOR CANCER, SPECIFICALLY SKIN CANCER. VESNA EXPLAINS NEW TREATMENTS AND JUST HOW QUICKLY RESEARCH HAS ADVANCED OVER THE LAST FEW YEARS, GIVING US A BRIGHTER OUTLOOK ON THE FUTURE OF CANCER TREATMENT.

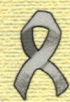
WALKIRIA WAS DIAGNOSED WITH A BRAIN TUMOUR IN 2018 AND HER STORY IS A COLLABORATION BETWEEN HERSELF AND HER DAUGHTER, ASHLING, WHO CONTINUES WALKIRIA'S STORY AND SHOWS JUST HOW LOVED AND APPRECIATED WALKIRIA WAS IN HER LIFETIME. WITHOUT WALKIRIA THIS ANTHOLOGY WOULDN'T EXIST.

THANK YOU ALL FOR YOUR HELP AND WISDOM IN BRINGING THIS PROJECT TO LIFE.

THE MAKING OF
"LIVING WITH CANCER: OUR STORIES"

COMICS ARE MUCH MORE THAN JUST PUTTING PEN TO PAPER, THERE ARE A VARIETY OF STEPS INVOLVED FROM HEARING A STORY TO CREATING PAGES. TO TURN OUR PARTICIPANTS STORIES INTO COMICS, WE – ASHLING AND CAT – TOOK THE INDIVIDUAL INTERVIEWS AND TRANSCRIBED THEM INTO SCRIPTS WE COULD THEN PASS ONTO OUR ARTISTS. IT WAS VERY IMPORTANT THAT EACH PERSON WAS SATISFIED WITH HOW THEIR STORY WAS WORDED AND HOW IT WOULD BE DRAWN WHICH INVOLVED A LITTLE BACK AND FORTH BETWEEN OURSELVES AND THEM. ONCE APPROVED, THE SCRIPTS INCLUDING PANEL NUMBERS, SPEECH BUBBLES AND SUGGESTED IMAGERY WERE ALL PASSED ONTO THE ARTISTS TO BEGIN MAKING THE STRIPS. WE ALSO MADE SURE TO INCLUDE NOTES TO PERSONALISE THE COMICS, SUCH AS THE STORYTELLERS FAVOURITE COLOURS AND SMALL DETAILS THAT WERE IMPORTANT TO THEM AND THEIR JOURNEY.

Carly's Story – Bright Smiles

Note 1: For security & privacy reasons, there are no reference photos of child patients or their families, and there are limited photos of the nursing staff that Carly works alongside, so for every character that is not Carly, feel free to improvise on their character design.

Page 1
Leave space at the top of this page for the comic title & credits.

Panel 1: Carly in her nurse's uniform, in the background there is a backdrop of London – the London Eye, Big Ben, etc.
Carly: Hi there, my name is Carly! I'm a Band 5 childrens nurse in bone marrow transplant. I've been working in London for 2 and a half years.

Panel 2: An empty yellow room with big windows, the lighting is dim and it's raining outside. There are some kids toys – teddy bears, building blocks, alphabet blocks and so on – strewn about the floor. The toys aren't damaged; it looks like they've barely been played with.
Caption: Working in the Children's cancer unit, people might assume the worst – that it's a sad place, that nobody survives, or that all we nurses do is just play all day with the children.

Panel 3: The same room as in the last panel, but the room is full of life; outside it's sunny and there are stickers of unicorns, cute bugs and other animals & cutouts of flower paintings on the window. The kids are playing with the toys; one nurse is playing with one of the children, one nurse is sitting and taking notes on a large (thick) clipboard, and another nurse is helping a young child to eat.
Caption: But the truth is that the ward is full of hope, laughter and joy!

Panel 4: Just a panel with Carly speaking. Use a flat colour (turquoise or yellow) for the background.
Carly: As a nurse, playing with the children is certainly one of the perks of the job, but we do so much more than that.

Panel 5: A large panel (either wide, tall or both) to fit 3 scenes in one; 1) A nurse changing a baby's nappy. 2) A nurse sitting beside an older child, reading & showing them the contents of a maths textbook while the child looks like they're thinking and writing in a school book on top of the over-bed table attached to their bed – there are other books on the bed and maybe on the over-bed table as well. 3) A nurse brushing another childs teeth.
Caption: Care for the children at the ward is 24/7 – We take care of their hygiene needs, education and oral care, and that's just one aspect of the work.

Naomi's Story Take Your Time

Note 1: Naomi's blog where she recorded a lot of her feelings on treatment is called *raindrops to ripples* so if raindrop/ripple motifs can be incorporated into panelling that would be a nice callback to that. Don't feel the need to force it however!
Note 2: Please refer to the descriptive references as well as photo references. All references will be labeled appropriately in relation to the part of the script it is needed for.

Page 1
Leave enough space at the top of this page for the comic title & credits.

Panel 1: Naomi is in a fox onesie, relaxing and looking peaceful with a cup of tea while writing something in a journal. Panel 2 depicts the scene she's writing about which could either fade into panel 1 or have more of a solid border (artist discretion).
Caption: April 1st, 2016.

Panel 2: Naomi is with her family, speaking with a Doctor. See reference image for the lay-out of the room & placement of everyones seats.
Doctor: We have your results, Naomi. It's Cancer. Grade II Astrocytoma in the brain.

Panel 3: Close up of Naomi's face looking pensive/scared.
Naomi, thinking: This is the worst April Fool's joke ever.

Panel 4: (maybe multiple shots with the narration over the top): Visuals of Naomi's hands clutching a small stone which has the soft shape of a love-heart, rolling it around in her hands. It's a wishing stone, marbling & grey.
Caption: I was diagnosed with a brain tumour on the right side of my brain in the front of the motor cortex in 2016, at only 20 years old. My life was changed completely from then on.

WHEN IT CAME TO THE CREATION OF THE PAGES, THE ARTISTS SENT US SNIPPETS OF THEIR PROGRESS WHICH WE WOULD SEND BACK OVER TO THE RELEVANT STORYTELLERS FOR FEEDBACK AND FURTHER EDITS. WE WANTED TO MAKE SURE THAT THE ARTISTS WERE ABLE TO EASILY INCLUDE THEIR PERSONAL CREATIVE FLAIR TO THE PAGES AS WELL, SO NOTES ON THEIR CREATIVE CHOICES WERE ALSO SENT BACK TO THE STORYTELLERS. WE WOULD ALSO USE THEIR FEEDBACK TO WORK OUT SPACING FOR TEXT AND OTHER EDITORIAL ELEMENTS ON OUR END.

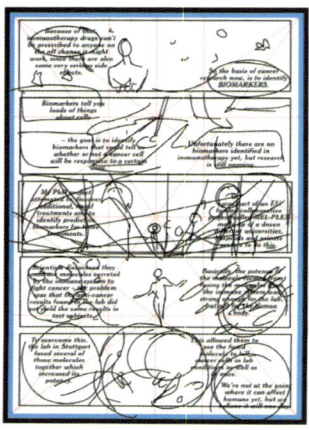 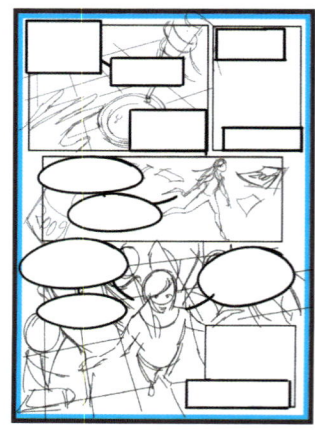 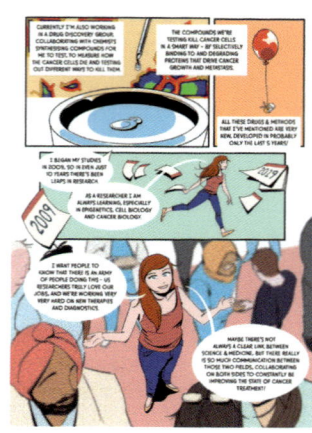

COLLABORATION WAS KEY IN THIS PROJECT, AND THAT EXTENDED TO THE ILLUSTRATION WORK AS WELL. HERE'S ONE EXAMPLE OF THIS: SARAH HOLLIDAY'S ILLUSTRATION WENT THROUGH A LOT OF CHANGES – FOLLOWING FEEDBACK FROM US, SHE MADE EDITS SUCH AS ALTERING COMPOSITION, TEXT SIZE, AND THE FINAL COLOUR CHOICES. WHILE WE LOVED ALL THE COLOUR OPTIONS, WE UNANIMOUSLY CHOSE THE BLUE + PINK COLOUR SCHEME BECUASE IT ENVOKES FEELINGS OF CALMNESS. GETTING THE RIGHT ATMOSPHERE FOR EACH PIECE OF ARTWORK WAS VERY IMPORTANT!

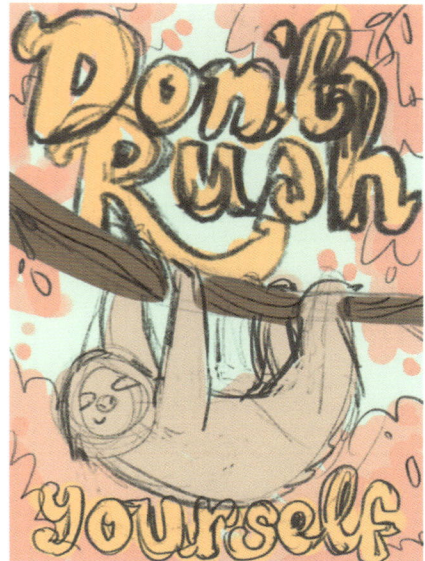
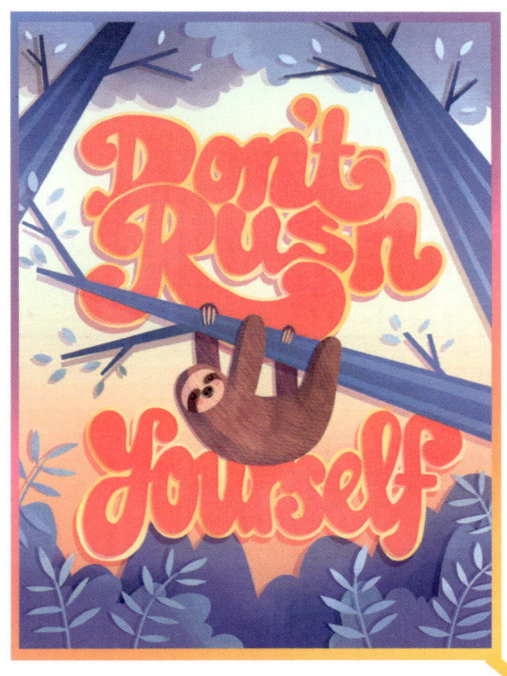
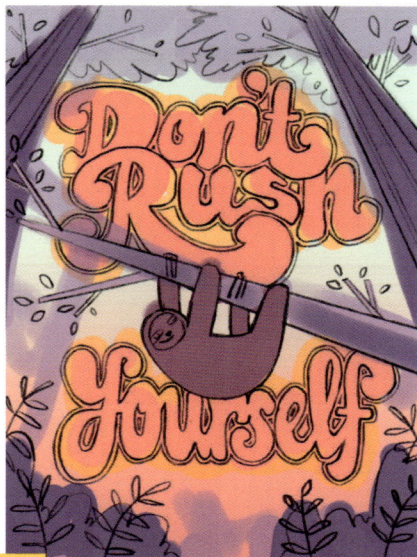
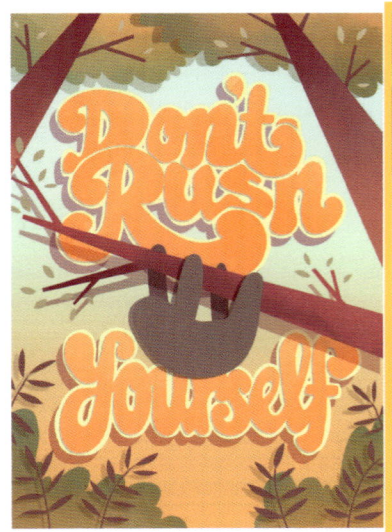
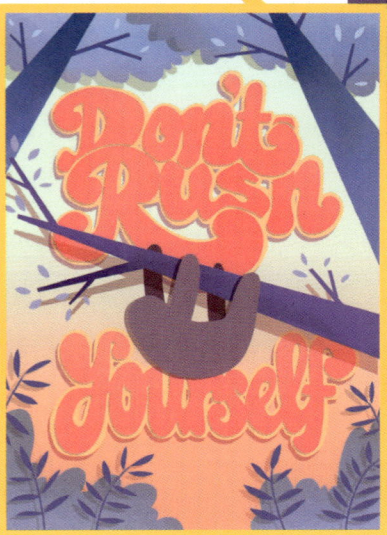
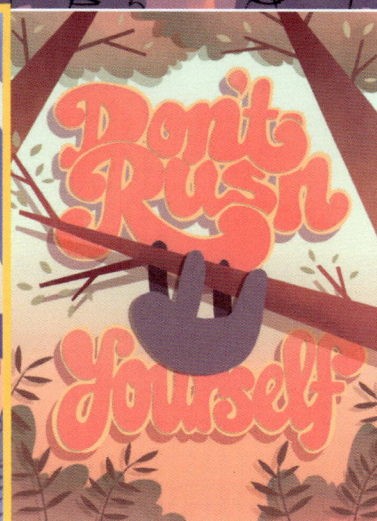

THIS PROJECT WOULD NOT HAVE BEEN POSSIBLE WITHOUT THE GENEROUS DONATIONS FROM OUR KICKSTARTER BACKERS:

ABI
ABI COOPER
ADAM BALSON
ADAM IAN BARRY
ALANNA BUTCHART
ALEX LOADER
ALEXANDRE CORBINEAU
ALEXIS M ORTIZ PEREZ
ALLY P
AMANDA KEEN
AMBER CANTIN
AMELIA IKEDA
AMY LOUISE MCCOULL
ANDREW BEAN
ANDY BRIDGE
ANNA LAU
ANNA RICE
AOIFE
ARMANDO WILDERMAN
BHP COMICS
BEE
BERNIE
BOB QUEK
BRETT MURRAY
BRIAN TYRRELL
BRITISHMUFFIN
C.L. FONTANA
CALUM LAIRD
CAROLINE CLUTTERBUCK
CASH O.
CAT DENNIS
CATARINA HENRIQUE
CHERYL FISHER
CHRIS & BECKY Z
CHRISTIAN REINHARDT
CHRISTINE O'DELL
CHRISTOPHER KUSH
CLIFF BALSON
COUNTWAY LIBRARY
CRAIG PATON
CURTIS JEWELL
DALLAN

DANIEL CROWLEY
DANIEL VERBIT
DARIA BARTOSIEWICZ
DAVID SMITH
DENISE LAFFERTY
DEVIN CONNELLY
DIVYA JINDAL-SNAPE
DONNA CHESHIRE
DYLAN
ELDRICH SOLMEYER
ELLY GLADMAN
EMIL N. TÓT
EMMY MADDY JOHNSTON
ERIN KEEPERS
ERIN SUBRAMANIAN
EVERSONG
FERMIN SERENA HORTAS
FRANCES BROWN
GARY ROBERTSON
GERARD LARKIN
GIORGIA DEL VERME
GORDON SHAW
HAILEY AUSTIN
HANNAH H
HANNAH MUIR
HANNAH TAYLOR
HARRY SAXON
HEALTHCARE FUTURISTS
HEATHER STEWART
HOLLY JONES
JACK VIRTUE
JACQUI BAIGENT
JANE WHITMAN
JARED BLUMBERG
JASMIN BONILLA
JASON CRASE
JEFFREY RADLOFF
JHOUSTONRITCHIE
JOCE KOFKE
JOE ROMERO
JOHN STEWART CAMPBELL
JOHN TAYLOR

THIS PROJECT WOULD NOT HAVE BEEN POSSIBLE WITHOUT THE GENEROUS DONATIONS FROM OUR KICKSTARTER BACKERS:

JOMIO & RUELIETE
JUDY VERNON
JULIE
JULIET MCMULLIN
JUSTIINA LEHTINEN
KAI SHAPARD
KATHARINE HUNT
KATHY KROMM
KATHRYN GARNIER
KAY KITCHING
KEILIDH BRADLEY
KEITH BACON
KELLY WYETH
LAURA BROWN
LAURA DAVIDSON
LAUREN MCLAUGHLIN
LENKA GLYNN-HAVEL
LIAM OSTLERE
LIDDY LAIRD
LORNA FOSTER
LOUISE KIRBY
MAGGIE MCCABE
MAIRI CLAIRE HUBBARD
MAJELLA MCCOY
MARK SUTHERLAND
MARKO FLEMING
MARTINA BACON
MATHIEU BOUCKAERT
MATTHEW B
MATTHEW BECKHAM
MATTHEW HARDY
MAURICE SMITH
MAYCONTAINHYJINKS
MCKAYS
MEGAN COTTER
MELANIE
MELANNIE HERNANDEZ
MELINDA NGUYEN
MICHI
MIKE
MILLIE MACKIE
MILMO

MIMZEE BREWER
MONICA WHEELER
NATALIA MYSZAK
OLIVIA HICKS
OLIVIA MCELVANEY
P. F. ANDERSON
PARKER RYDON
PATE MCKISSACK
PAUL GRAVETT
PAULA MEIRELES
PIA BLUME
RACHEL H SANDERS
RAJENDRA PISAVADIA
RAPHAEL
REBECCA OLLERTON
RHYS
RODDY AND JO OSTLERE
RON "CREWYLOU" EVANS
RONNIE GREENWOOD
ROSEALEE
SALLY LARKIN
SANDRA LEAHY
SAOIRSE MAHON
SARAH MEE
SEUMIDH MACDONALD
SHANNON COOKE
SHEENA CAMERON
SHIRLEY BLAIR
SINEAD
STEPHANIE BAZELEY
SUSAN WHYTE
SWORDFIRE
SYLPHIS
TASNEEM AHMED
THE MELT THE FLY BOYS
TONY BACON
VICKY STEPHEN
WILLIAM POTTER
ZACH OWEN
ZANAMEE
ZU DOM

THANK YOU.

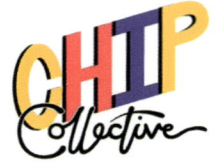